Eternal Flames

DEDICATION

To the man who lights me up every single day

-

This book was made possible by the delectable Raven who reawakened my stagnant energetic channels and reminded me of the deliciousness of living an orgasmic life

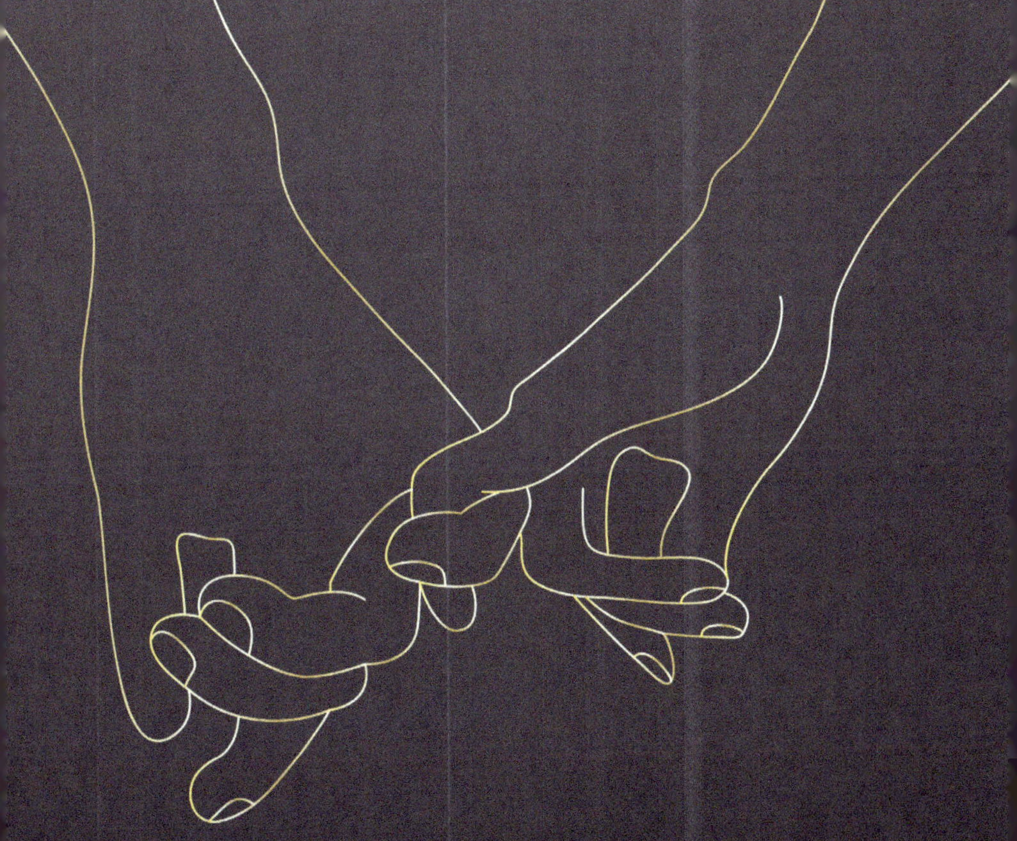

Eternal Flames

Eternal Flames
Eternal Flames

Foreword

This book came about after a beautfiul tantric reawakening,
and while I had previsously enjoyed the bountiful gifts of tantric
practice as a single, my partner was new to the delights.
In the proces of looking for beginner techniques, I found plenty
of instruction manuals, but no stories. No stories that allowed me
to imagine myself in the moment, no stories that explained the
wholeness of living a tantric life.

This work is a complete fiction, bearing no resemblance to my life
and not based specifically on people I know.

Where it does cross over into reality is by exploring the themes
common to many couples who engage in sacred sexuality and
tantric techniques, the pleasures and challenges of
non-monogamy, along with the more typical aspects of a
couples life.

with much love,
Linda x

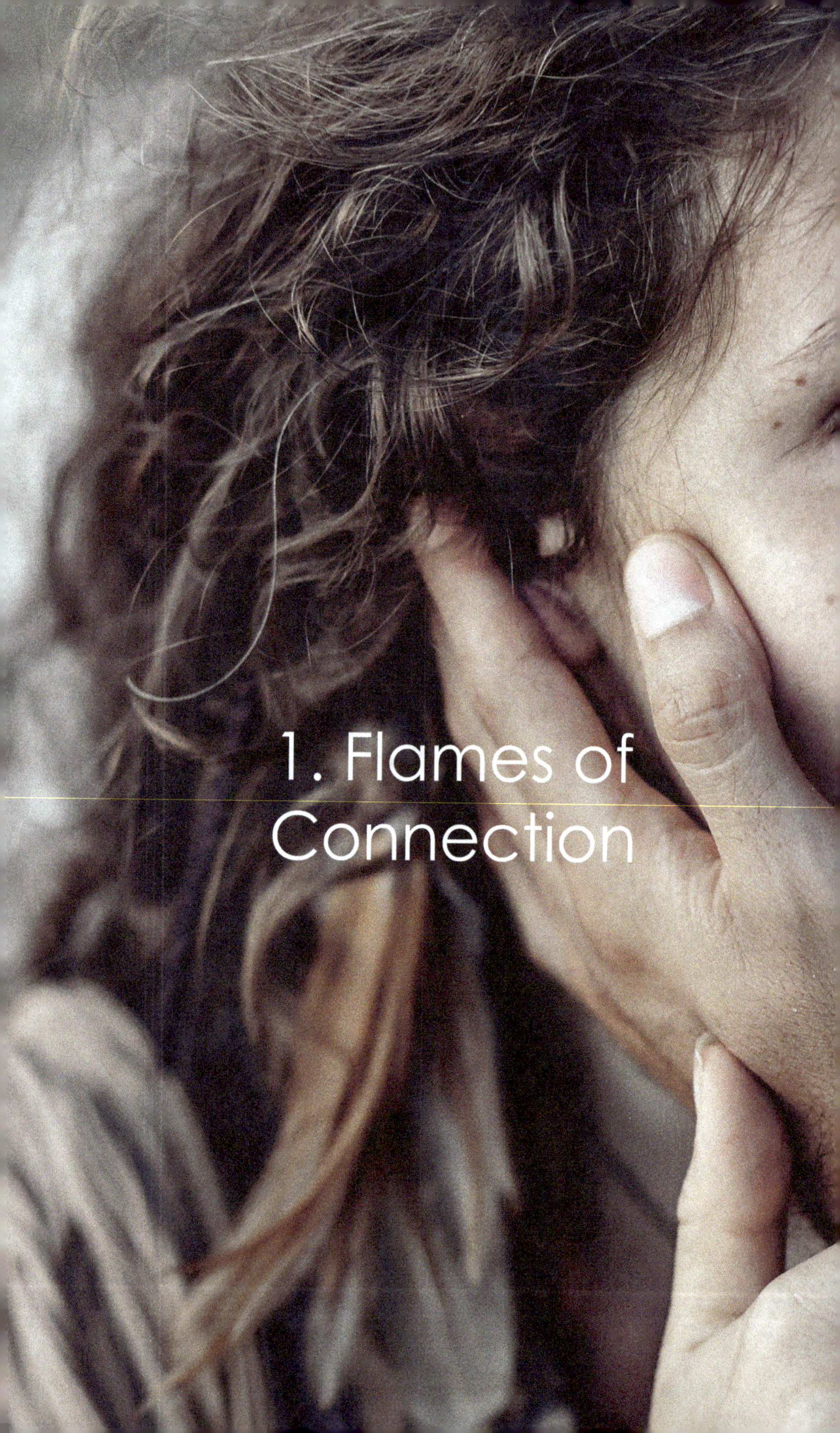
1. Flames of
Connection

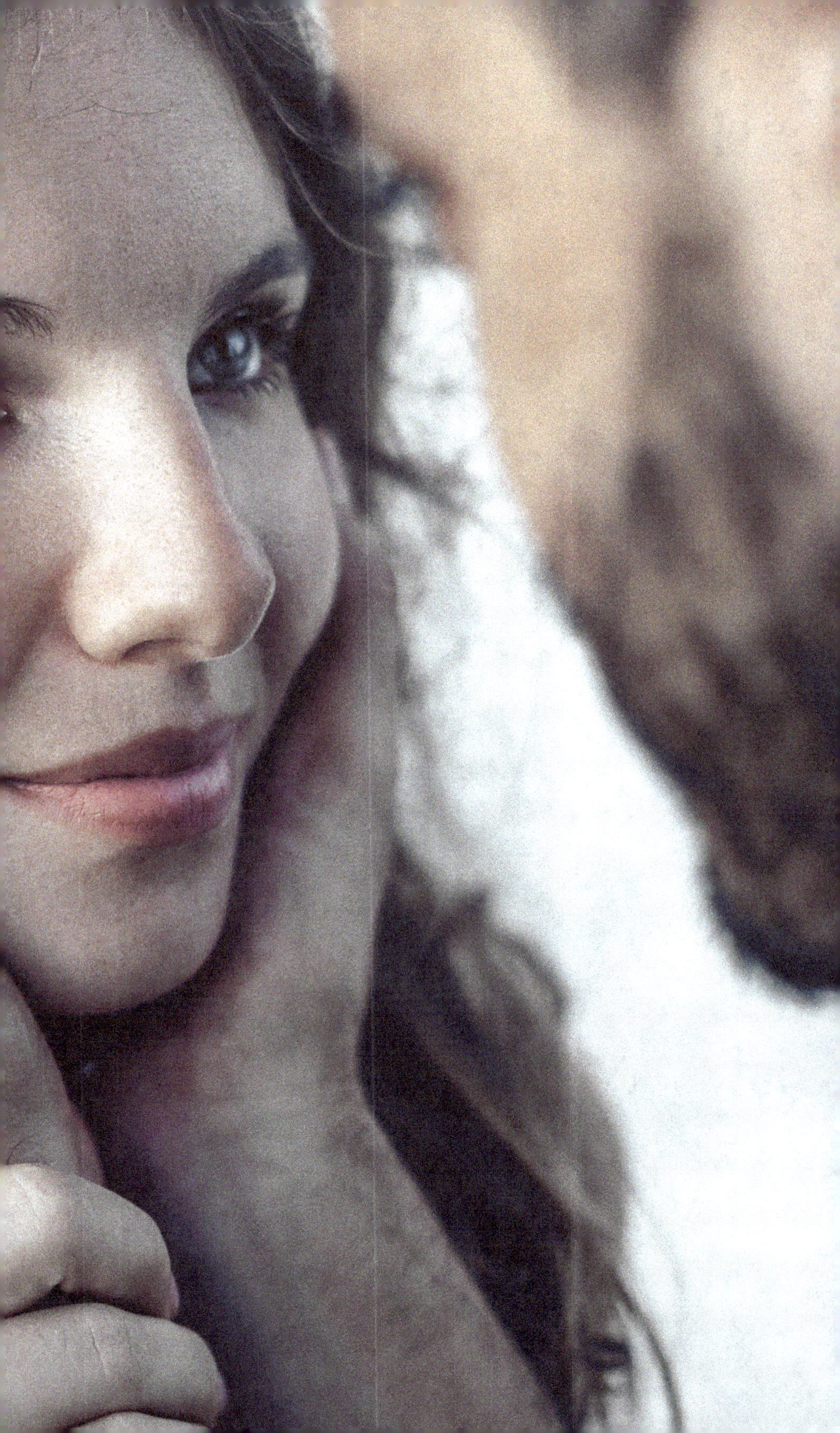

Chapter 1: Flames of Connection

The warm glow of the fireplace in Ethan's cosy living room cast dancing shadows on the walls, filled with books and memories. Mia, tall and slender, with her honey-coloured hair cascading over her shoulders, sat on a soft cushion, her gentle green eyes reflecting the flickering light. Ethan, his muscular frame relaxed yet poised, stoked the fire, his dark brown eyes glancing towards Mia with a mix of anticipation and nervousness.

Ethan's home, a charming, off-grid caretaker's cottage on the Mornington Peninsula, felt like a haven away from the world. The evening had unfolded beautifully after their dinner - laughter, shared stories, and a sense of growing intimacy. But now, as the embers crackled and whispered secrets to the night, Ethan proposed something new, something different – a tantric ritual.

Mia's initial reaction was one of uncertainty. Her past, marred by a toxic relationship, had made her cautious. Ethan's description of the ritual, though well-intentioned, had sounded more arcane than intimate. Sensing her hesitation, Ethan quickly reassured her, "It's not what it sounds like, I promise. It's about connection, about being present with each other. Nothing more."

He explained again, more simply this time, his voice a soothing balm. The ritual was a series of steps, he said, designed to foster a deeper, more spiritual connection. No pressure, no expectations – just two souls exploring the realms of emotional intimacy. Mia, touched by his sincerity and the evident depth of his feelings, agreed to give it a try.

They began in silence, preparing their space with care. Ethan lit a candle, its flame casting a soft, inviting glow. They sat facing each other, the heat from the fire mingling with the cool autumn air.

Ethan guided Mia through the breathing synchronisation. Their breaths, initially out of sync, soon found a harmonious rhythm. Mia felt her body relax; her mind clearing of distractions. There was something surprisingly calming about this shared act of breathing.

As they placed their hands over their hearts, Mia felt a warmth spreading through her chest. When Ethan tentatively reached out to place his hand over her heart, she welcomed the gesture. His touch was gentle, respectful. She could feel his heartbeat, strong and steady, a counterpoint to her own.

The eye gazing was the most intense part. At first, Mia's eyes darted away, unaccustomed to such direct, unguarded contact. But as she met Ethan's gaze, something shifted. His eyes were like pools of understanding and kindness, inviting her to let go of her fears. In that moment, they communicated more than words ever could. Mia felt seen, truly seen, in a way she had never experienced before.

Chanting the mantra, their voices merged into a single, harmonious vibration. The sound "Om" resonated in the room, enveloping them in a shared energy. Mia felt connected not just to Ethan, but to something larger, something profound.

In the silent appreciation that followed, Mia was acutely aware of every sensation – the warmth of the fire, the softness of the cushion beneath her, the gentle pressure of Ethan's hand still resting over her heart.
She felt a deep sense of peace, a connection that went beyond the physical.

As they concluded the ritual, their hands together in front of their hearts, Mia felt a surge of gratitude. Gratitude for this moment, for Ethan's gentle guidance, for the unexpected journey they had embarked upon together.

Ethan blew out the candle, the smoke curling up and vanishing into the night. As he turned to Mia, their eyes locked, and she saw in his gaze a reflection of her own feelings – a desire to explore this connection further, to see where this path of emotional and spiritual intimacy might lead.

They had started the evening as two individuals, each with their own histories and hesitations. But as the fire died down to glowing coals, they sat together, united by an experience that was as profound as it was unexpected. In the sacred space they had created, a new flame had been kindled – a flame that promised to light their way forward, together.

Tantric Ritual for Beginners

A simple and gentle 15 minute ritual designed for beginners in tantric practice. This ritual can be practised alone or with a partner. Approach with an open heart and mind, be present and respectful throughout the process.

Total Duration: 15 minutes

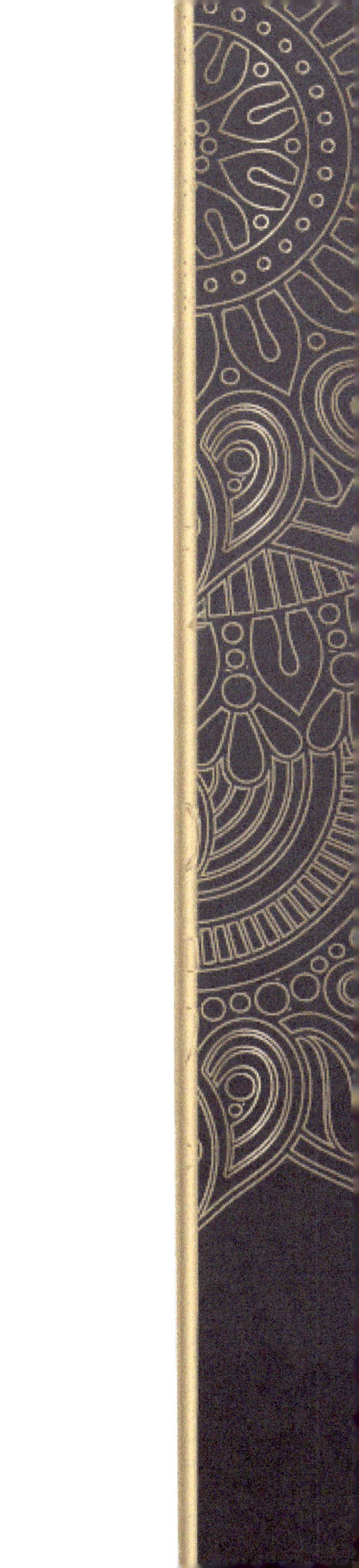

Preparation:
Find a comfortable quiet space where you won't be
disturbed.
Sit on a cushion or mat, maintaining a comfortable posture.
If with a partner, sit facing each other, with your hands on
your own knees.
Light a candle or incense to create a serene ambiance.

Breathing Synchronisation (3 minutes):
Close your eyes and take deep, slow breaths.
If with a partner, try to synchronise your breathing. Inhale
and exhale together to create a rhythm.
Focus on the sound and feel of your breath, letting go of
other thoughts.

Heart-Centred Connection (3 minutes):
Place your right hand over your heart and your left hand
over it.
If with a partner, after a moment, extend your right hand to
your partner's heart, keeping your left hand on your own.
Feel the warmth of your hands and the beat of the heart,
either yours or your partner's.

Eye Gazing (2 minutes):
Open your eyes and gently gaze into your own or your
partner's eyes.
Maintain a soft gaze, avoiding staring. It's about
connecting, not intimidating.
If thoughts arise, gently bring your focus back to the eyes.

Silent Appreciation (2 minutes):
Sit in silence, appreciating the moment.
Reflect on the feelings of peace, connection, and love.
If with a partner, acknowledge your gratitude for their
presence and energy.

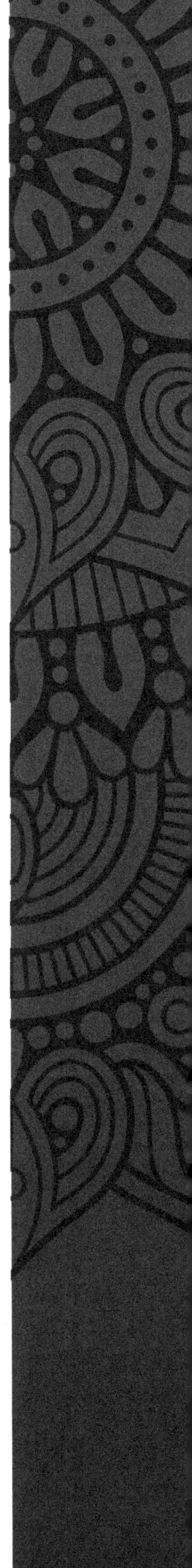

Eternal Flames

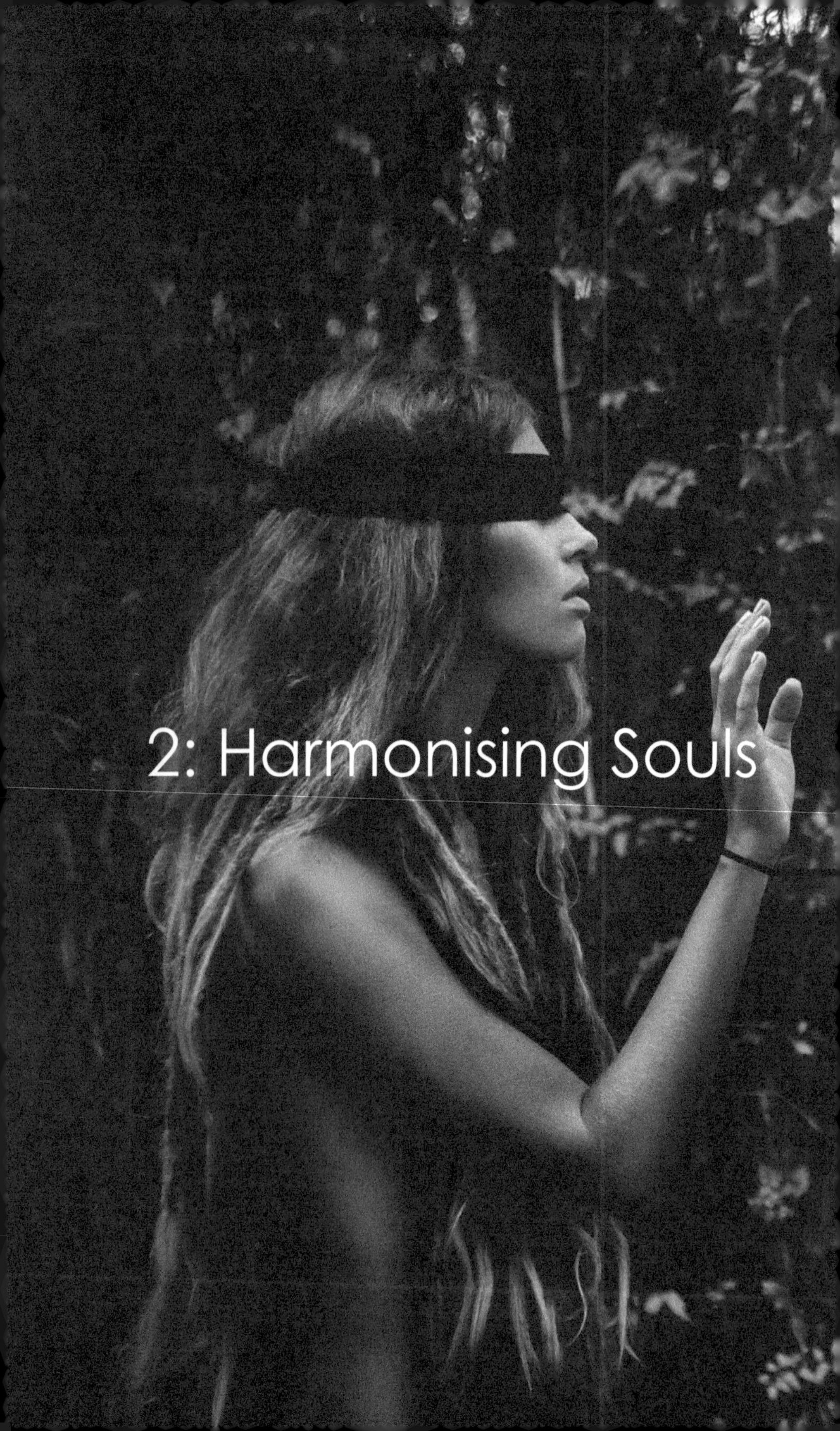

2: Harmonising Souls

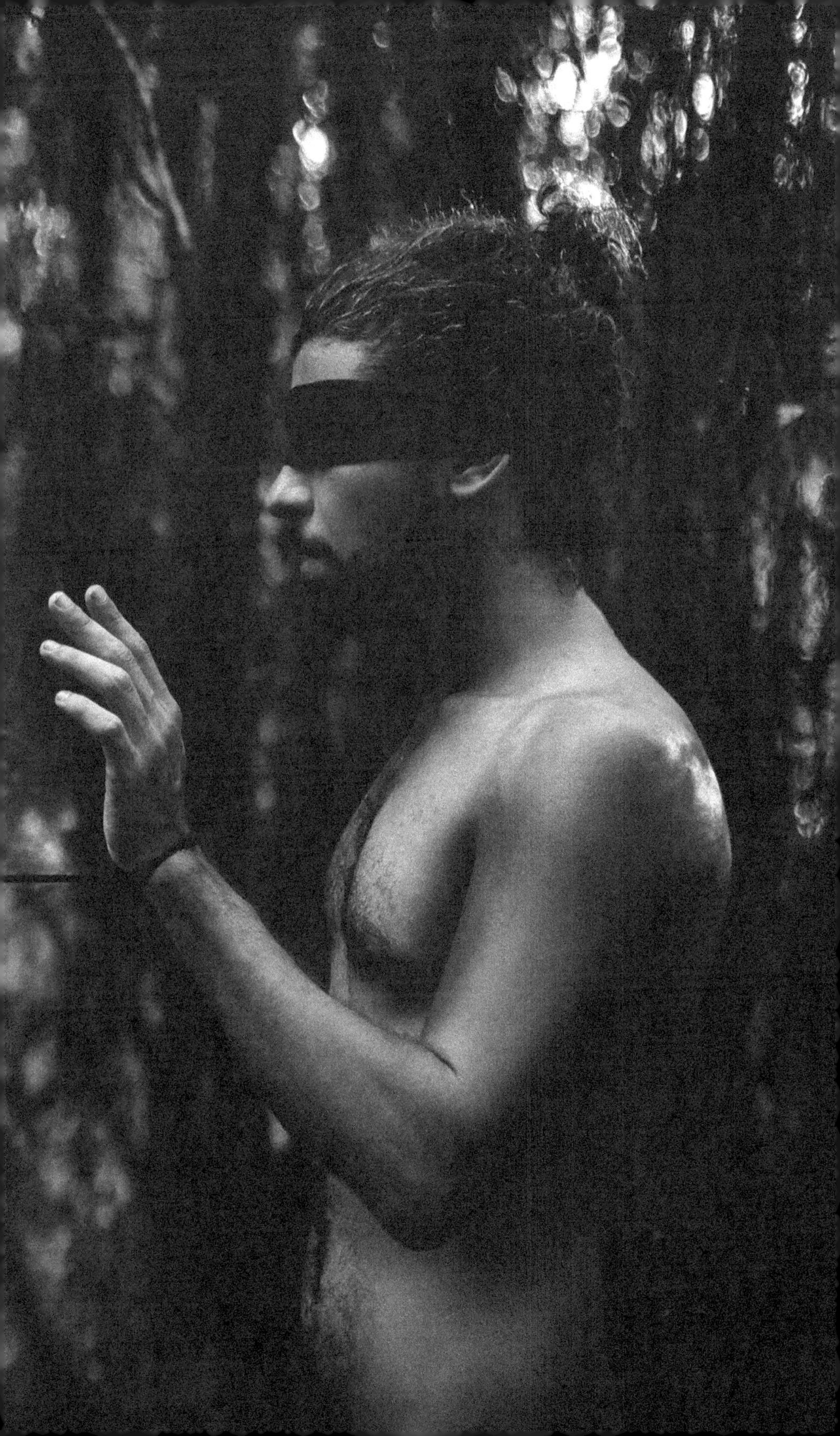

Chapter 2: Harmonising Souls

Six months had woven Mia and Ethan closer, threading their lives into a tapestry rich with love, understanding and a shared journey of discovery. Their relationship, once tentative and cautious, now thrived with the depth of a committed, loving bond.
This evening, as the autumn leaves whispered secrets to the wind outside, they prepared to embark on a new chapter of their spiritual journey together.

Ethan had transformed their living room into a sacred space. Candles flickered, casting a warm, inviting glow, and the scent of sandalwood incense filled the air. Mia, her long honey-coloured hair braided to the side, sat facing Ethan on a plush cushion. His dark eyes sparkled with excitement and a deep sense of serenity.

They began with grounding and centering, their breaths deep and synchronised. As they visualised roots extending from their root chakras and a beam of light connecting their crown chakras to the universe, a profound sense of connection to the earth and the cosmos enveloped them.

Moving into the chakra awareness and balancing, Ethan and Mia took turns sharing their thoughts and feelings about each chakra. They spoke of fears and dreams, of blockages and flows, their words weaving a tapestry of shared vulnerability and strength.

At the root chakra, Mia spoke of her growing sense of security with Ethan, her voice soft yet steady. Ethan, placing his hands gently near her base, chanted the Bija mantra 'LAM', his voice resonating with strength and support.

As they progressed upward, each chakra unraveled deeper layers of their personalities and their relationship. The sacral chakra revealed their desires and creativity, the solar plexus chakra their personal power and self-confidence, and the heart chakra, the epicentre of their love and compassion.

When they reached the throat chakra, Mia's voice wavered as she shared her struggle with expressing her deepest fears. Ethan listened, his eyes reflecting empathy and understanding. Chanting 'HAM' together, they sought to unlock and balance this

channel of communication.
The third eye chakra stirred visions of their shared future, dreams interlacing with a profound understanding. As they chanted 'OM', their voices harmonised, creating a vibration that seemed to echo through their very souls.

Finally, at the crown chakra, they sat in silent meditation, envisioning a radiant light that connected them to something greater than themselves. The mantra 'AH' floated in the air, a sound as light as the ether, binding their spirits in a moment of transcendental unity.

In the tantric breathing and energy exchange that followed, they sat in the Yab-Yum position, their breaths and hearts in perfect sync. They visualised an exchange of energies, a vibrant loop that flowed seamlessly between them, each inhale drawing in love and trust, each exhale releasing harmony and understanding.

As the meditation deepened, a golden light seemed to envelop them, a tangible manifestation of their combined energies. It was a dance of light and shadow, of giving and receiving, of two souls harmonising in a dance as old as time.

In the closing of the practice, they shared their experiences, their voices soft and reflective. Mia spoke of a profound sense of belonging, of being understood and cherished. Ethan expressed his awe at the depth of their connection, feeling as if their souls had been entwined not just for months, but for lifetimes.

They ended the ritual with a heartfelt embrace, a silent promise of more to explore and discover together. As they blew out the candles, the room didn't darken; instead, it seemed to retain a glow, the residual warmth of their shared energy.

This evening, in their sacred space, Mia and Ethan had not just harmonised their chakras; they had harmonised their souls. And in this harmonisation, they found not just love, but a profound and resounding peace.

Focusing on Chakras

This ritual is designed to deepen the connection between partners through energy work and mindfulness, enhancing both emotional and spiritual intimacy. It's important to approach each step with respect, presence and an open heart.

Total Duration: 15 minutes

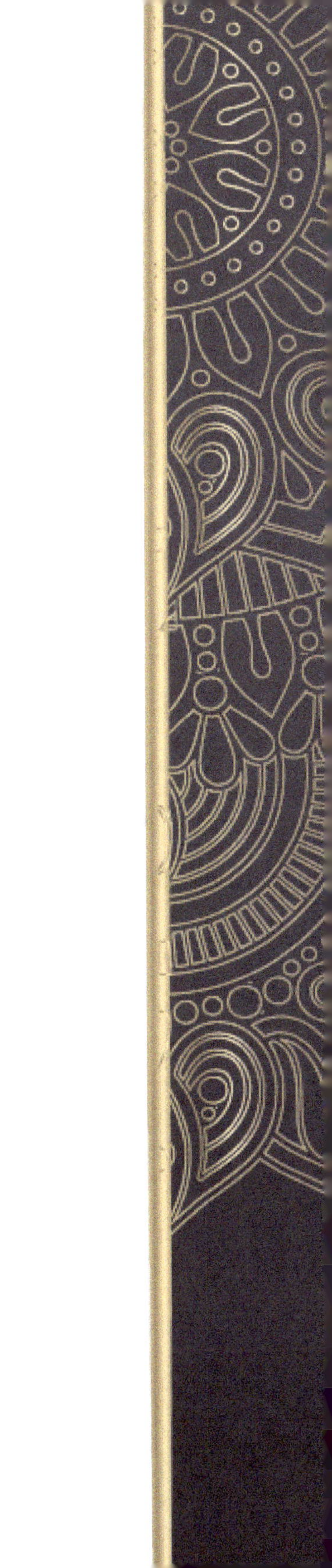

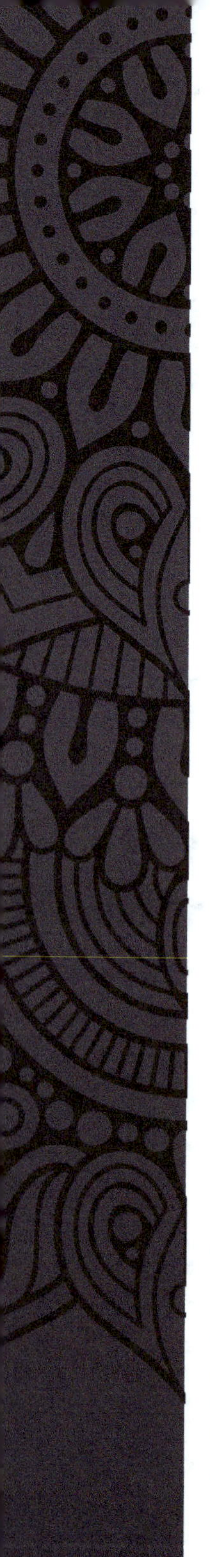

Preparation:
Create a sacred and comfortable space
Sit facing each other on cushions or mats in a quiet, peaceful room.
Light candles and incense to enhance the ambiance and signify the beginning of a sacred practice.

Grounding and Centring (5 minutes):
Begin by closing your eyes and taking deep, long breaths.
Visualise roots growing from the base of your spine (root chakra) into the earth, grounding you.
Imagine a beam of light from the crown of your head (crown chakra) connecting to the universe, centring you.

Chakra Awareness and Balancing (30 minutes):
Focus on each of the seven chakras, starting from the root chakra and moving up to the crown chakra.

For each chakra:
Share what each chakra represents to you and discuss any blockages or imbalances you might be feeling.

Place hands on or near the location of each chakra (without making physical contact if it's a private area).

Visualise the colour associated with each chakra and imagine energy flowing freely through it.

Chant the corresponding Bija mantras (LAM for Root, VAM for Sacral, RAM for Solar Plexus, YAM for Heart, HAM for Throat, OM for Third Eye, and AH for Crown) together to enhance the energy flow.

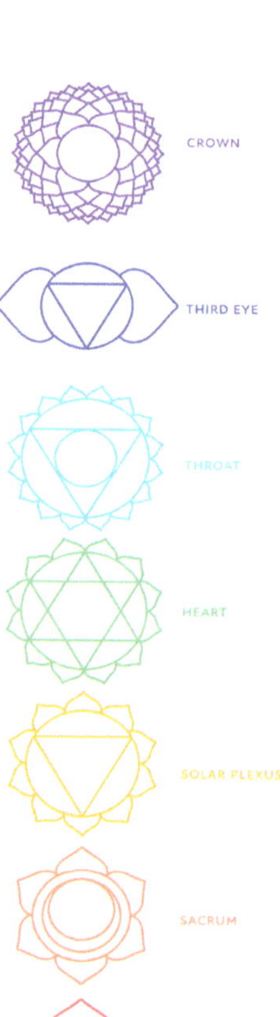

Tantric Breathing and Energy Exchange (10 minutes):
Sit very close to each other in Yab-Yum position (one
partner sitting on the other's lap) or a comfortable
alternative.
Practice deep, synchronised breathing.
Visualise drawing up your partner's energy with each
inhale and sending your energy to your partner with each
exhale, creating a circular energy flow between you.

Meditation and Visualisation (5-10 minutes):
Meditate together, visualising a harmonious blend of your
energies.
Visualise a golden light encompassing both of you,
symbolising unity, love, and spiritual connection.

Closing the Practice (5 minutes):
Share your experiences, feelings, and any insights that
arose during the practice.
Express gratitude towards each other for sharing this
spiritual journey.
Gently bring the practice to a close, perhaps with a bow or
a heartfelt embrace.

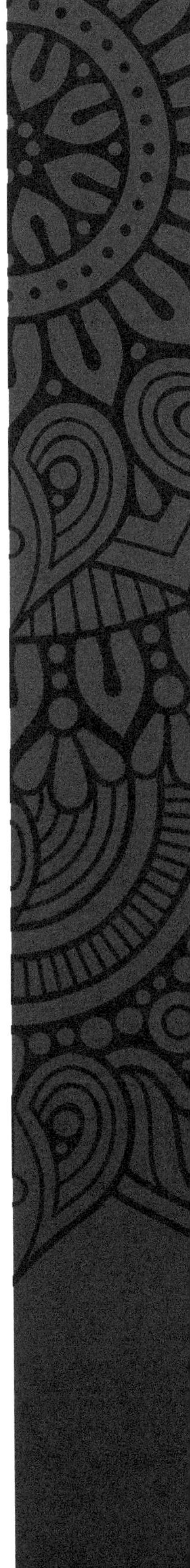

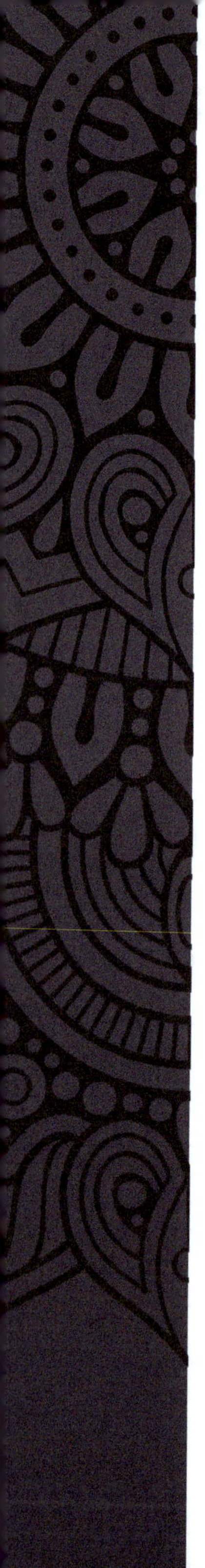

CROWN CHAKRA
SAHASRARA
"I UNDERSTAND"
Knowledge, Consciousness,
Fulfilment, Spirituality

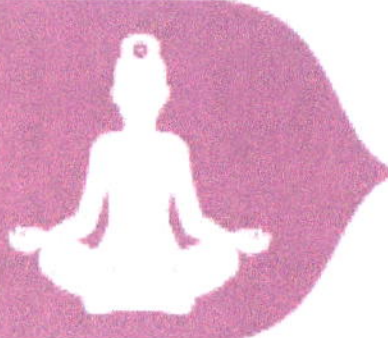

THIRD EYE CHAKRA
AJNA
"I SEE"
Intuition, Lucidity,
Meditation, Trust

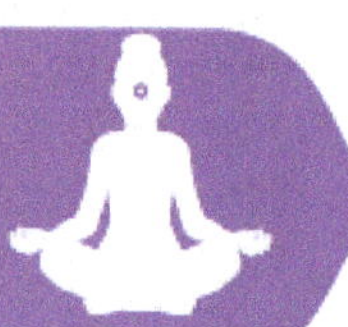

THROAT CHAKRA
VISHUDDHA
"I TALK"
Communication, Expression,
Creativity, Inspiration

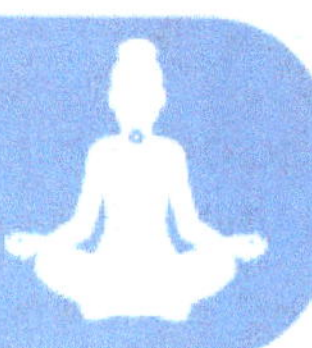

HEART CHAKRA
ANAHATA
"I LOVE"
Acceptance, Love,
Compassion, Sincerity

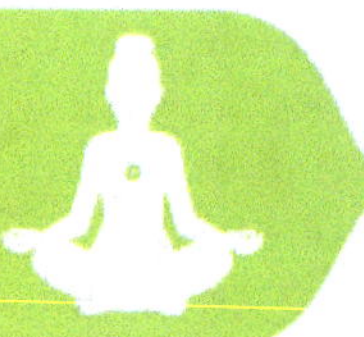

SOLAR PLEXUS CHAKRA
MANIPURA
"I DO"
Strength, Personality,
Power, Determination

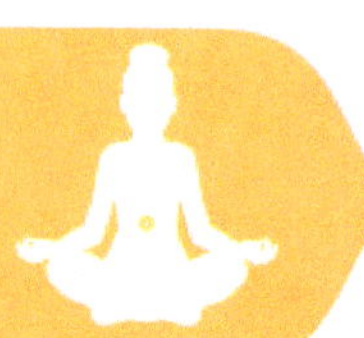

SACRAL CHAKRA
SVADHISTHANA
"I FEEL"
Sensuality, Sexuality,
Pleasure, Sociability

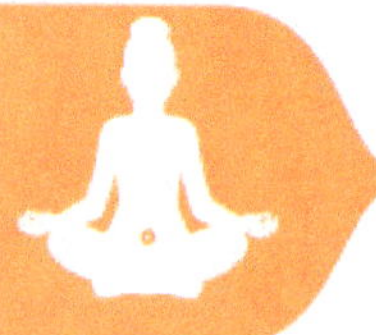

ROOT CHAKRA
MULADHARA
"I AM"
Energy, Stability,
Comfort, Safety

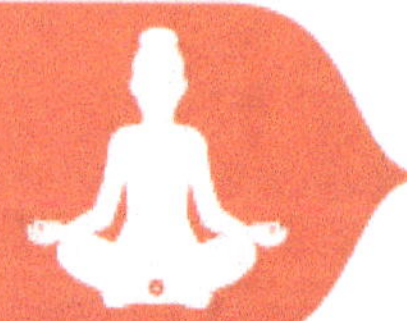

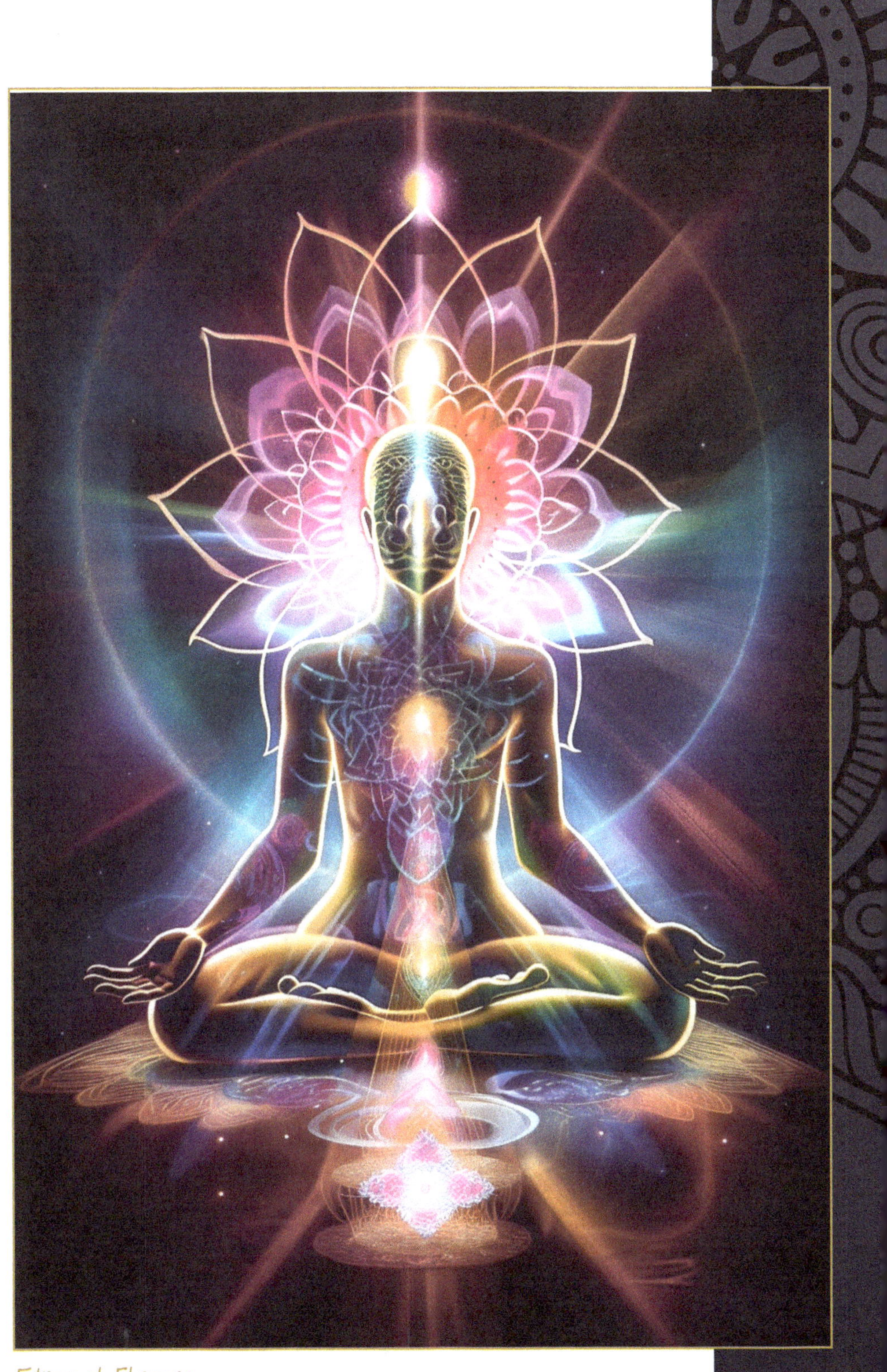

Eternal Flames

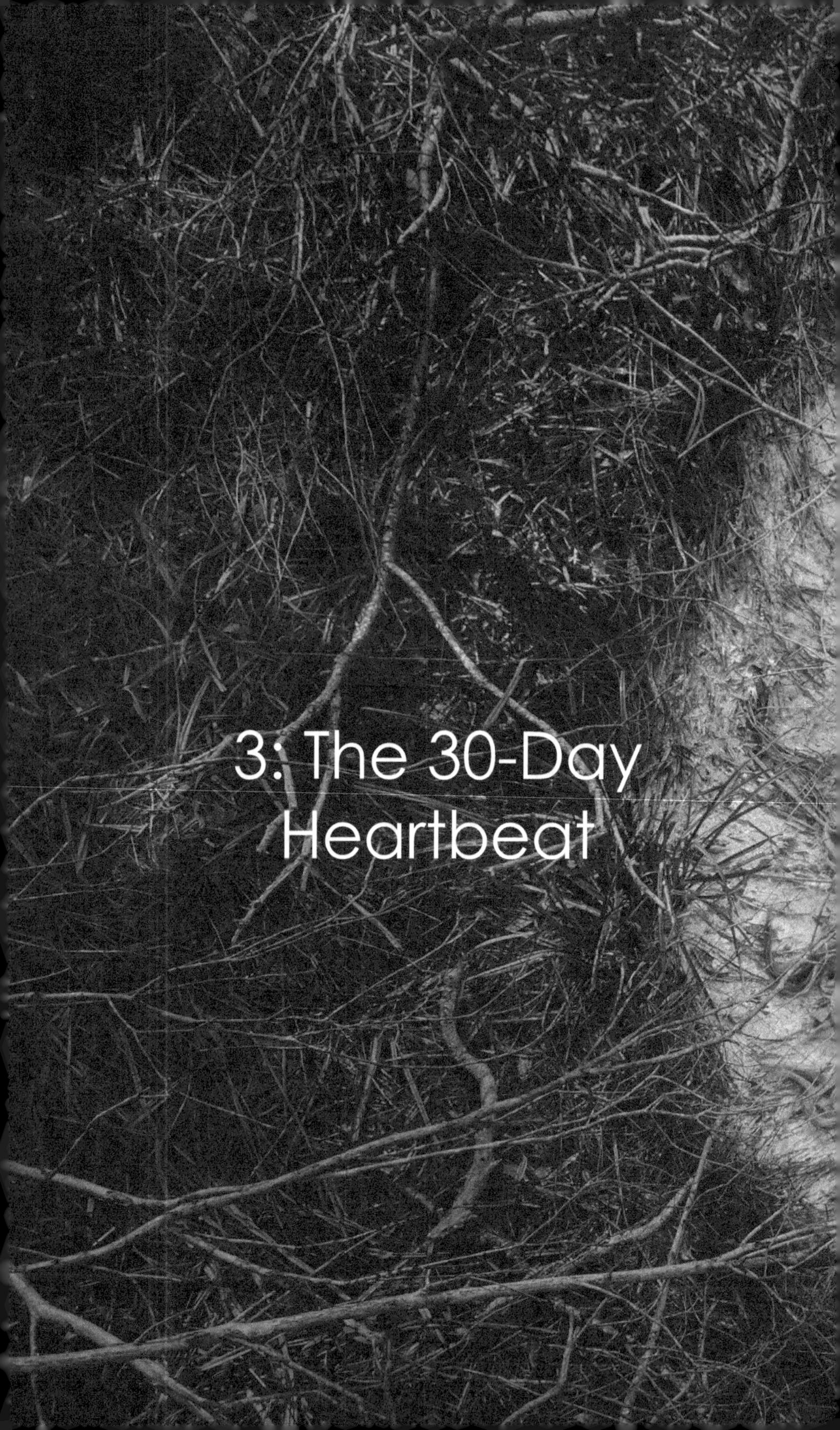
3: The 30-Day
Heartbeat

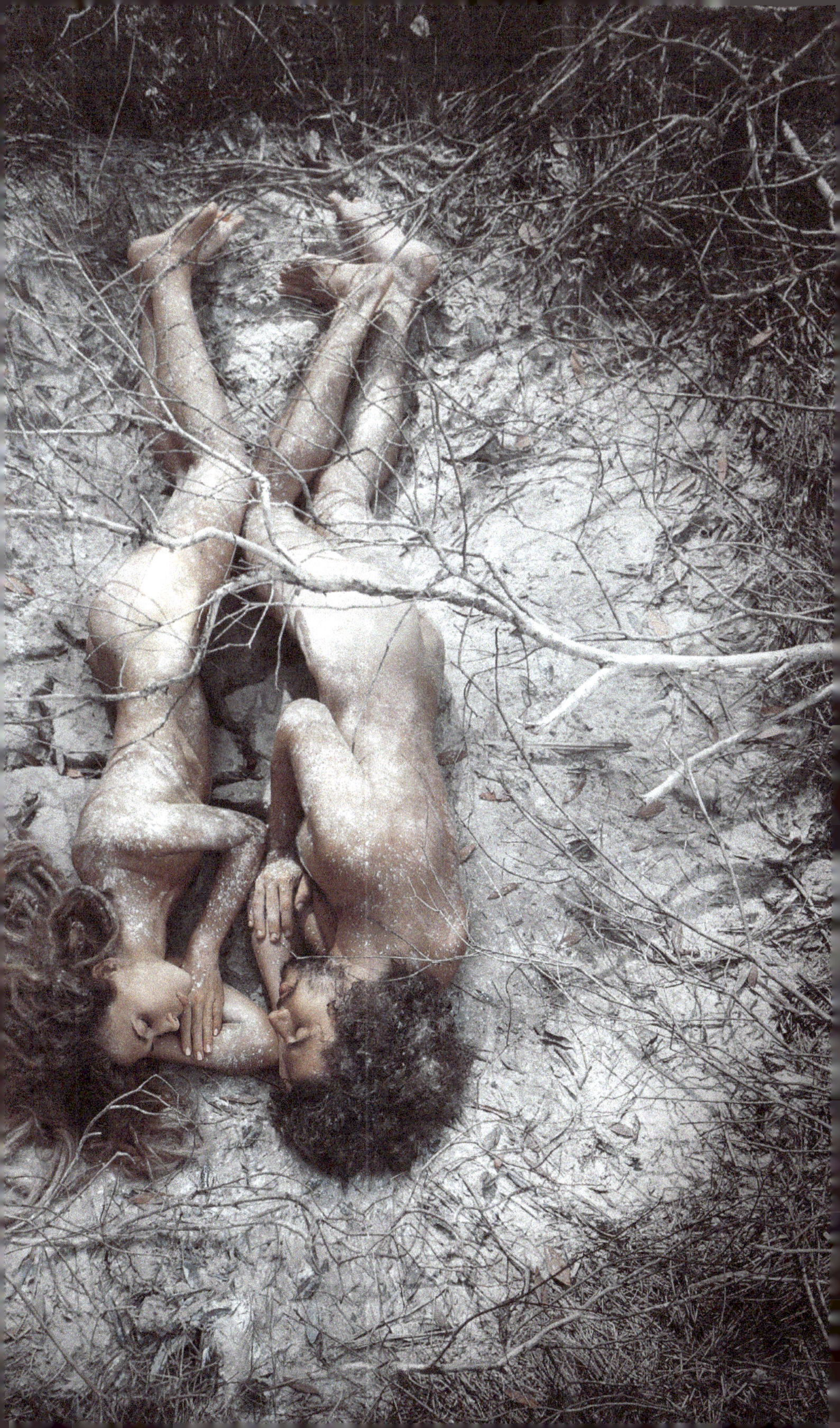

Chapter 3: The 30-Day Heartbeat

Two years into their journey together, Mia and Ethan's life at the cottage had blossomed into a beautiful, if sometimes hectic, shared existence. Between Mia's long hours at the veterinary clinic and Ethan's endless tasks in the vineyard, their moments of quiet togetherness had become rare treasures.

One evening, as they settled into the comfort of their living room, the fire crackling softly in the background, Mia shared something she had discovered: a 30-day tantra challenge. "It's just five minutes a day," she explained, her green eyes reflecting the firelight. "A way for us to reconnect, no matter how busy we are."

Ethan, always open to deepening their bond, agreed without hesitation. So, they began their new ritual, a commitment to each other and to the love that had grown between them.

On the first night, they sat facing each other, the familiarity of their ritual space wrapping around them like a warm embrace. They held hands, their fingers intertwining comfortably, as they closed their eyes and synchronised their breathing. In and out, their chests rose and fell together, a shared rhythm that instantly drew them closer, melting away the chaos of the day.

Next, they moved to the heart connection. Mia placed her hand over Ethan's heart, feeling its steady beat under her palm. Ethan mirrored her gesture, his hand warm over her heart. In that simple touch, they communicated love, appreciation, and a deep gratitude for each other's presence in their lives.

When they opened their eyes for the eye gazing, something magical happened. In Ethan's dark eyes, Mia saw not only her reflection but also the depth of their past two years - the joys, the challenges, and the growth. Ethan, gazing back, saw the same in Mia's bright eyes. No words were needed; their eyes spoke volumes, telling stories only they could understand.

As they concluded each session with expressions of gratitude, their words felt like gentle caresses, reaffirming their love and commitment. "I am grateful for your strength," Mia would say, or Ethan would whisper, "I cherish your kindness." Each affirmation was a seed planted, growing roots in their hearts.

Night after night, they met in their sacred space by the fire. Some nights were filled with laughter, others with tears, as they navigated the ebbs and flows of their shared life. But always, there was love - a steady, unbreakable bond that thrived under the nurturing of their daily practice.

As the 30 days came to an end, Mia and Ethan felt a renewed sense of closeness. The challenge had not only brought them together each day but had deepened their understanding and appreciation of each other. It was as if they had rediscovered a secret language, one spoken by hearts in harmony.

On the final night, as they completed their ritual, Mia leaned forward, her eyes sparkling with unshed tears of joy. "These five minutes with you," she said softly, "are the best part of my day." Ethan, his own eyes reflecting the same emotion, replied, "They're my heartbeat, Mia. You are my heartbeat."

In the gentle glow of the fire, in the cottage that had become their home, Mia and Ethan embraced, knowing that this ritual, these precious moments, would continue far beyond the 30 days.

For in those five minutes each day, they found not just love, but a reminder of why they had chosen each other, why they would always choose each other, every day, for all the days to come.

5 Minute Daily Tantric Practice

A simple and effective 5 minute daily tantric practice for couples. This ritual is designed to be easy to integrate into daily routines while still fostering a deep sense of connection and intimacy. Practice consistently for 30 days notice the strengthening emotional and spiritual bond between partners.

Total Duration: 5 minutes x 30 days

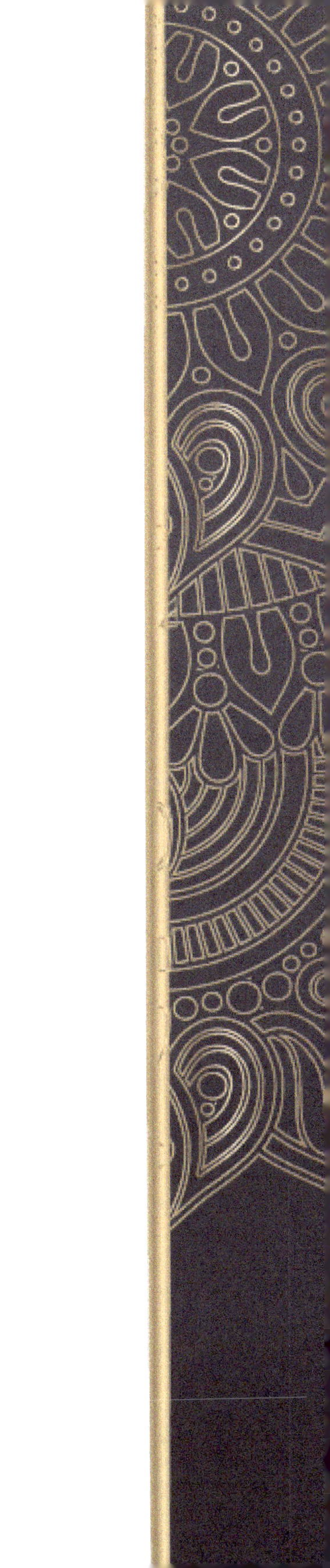

Preparation:
Find a quiet and comfortable space.
Stand, or sit facing each other on cushions or chairs, close
enough to hold hands.

Take a moment to acknowledge the commitment to this
daily practice and the presence of your partner.

Synchronised Breathing (1 minute):
Hold each other's hands and close your eyes.
Begin to breathe deeply and slowly, in unison. Inhale
together, then exhale together.
Focus on the rhythm of your combined breathing, feeling
the connection through your hands.

Heart Connection (1 minute):
Place your free hand over your own heart, then reach to
place your other hand over your partner's heart.
Feel the warmth of your hands and the heartbeat of your
partner.
Silently send thoughts of love and gratitude towards each
other.

Eye Gazing (1 minute):
Open your eyes and gaze softly into each other's eyes.
Maintain a gentle, loving gaze, without speaking.
Allow this eye contact to deepen your sense of connection
and understanding.

Closing with Gratitude (1 minute):
Share a brief statement of gratitude or affirmation with
each other. This could be as simple as "I am grateful for
you" or "I cherish our connection."
Conclude the practice with a gentle embrace or a kiss,
acknowledging the shared experience.
Take a deep breath together and then slowly release your
hands, carrying the sense of connection with you as you
transition back to your day.

30 Day Challenge

This challenge is for solo, couples or multi-partner practice.
Adjust the language to suit your needs.
The concept of this practice can also be adjusted and used with kids as a gratitude practice.

This practice can be a beautiful way to start or end the day, helping to maintain and deepen the bond between you and your partner.
Consistently dedicating these few minutes to each other every day will create a profound and lasting impact on your relationship.

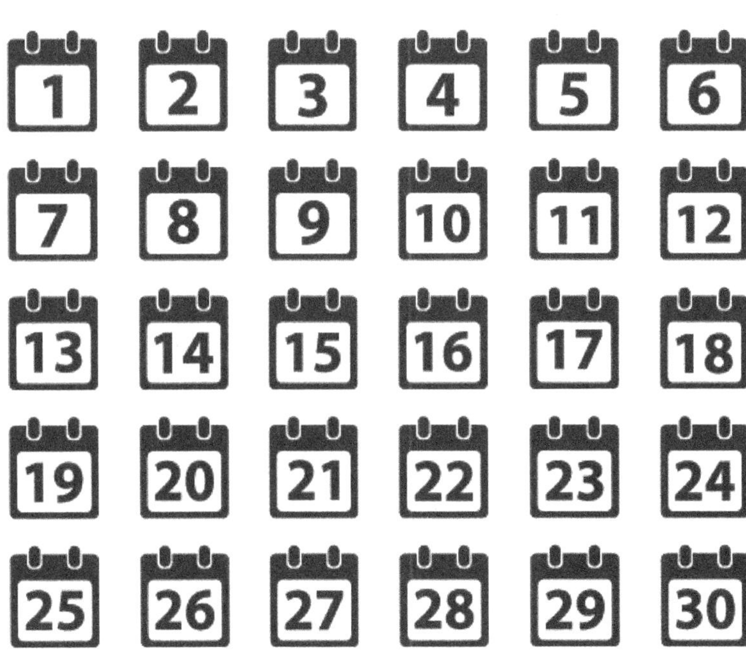

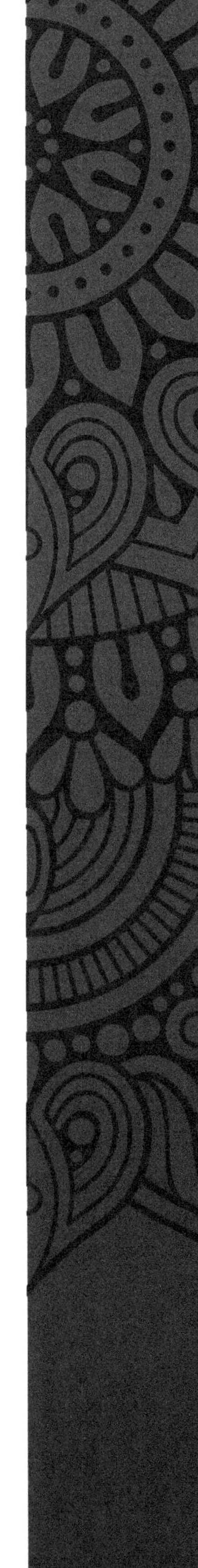

Eternal Flames

4: The Cacao Celebration

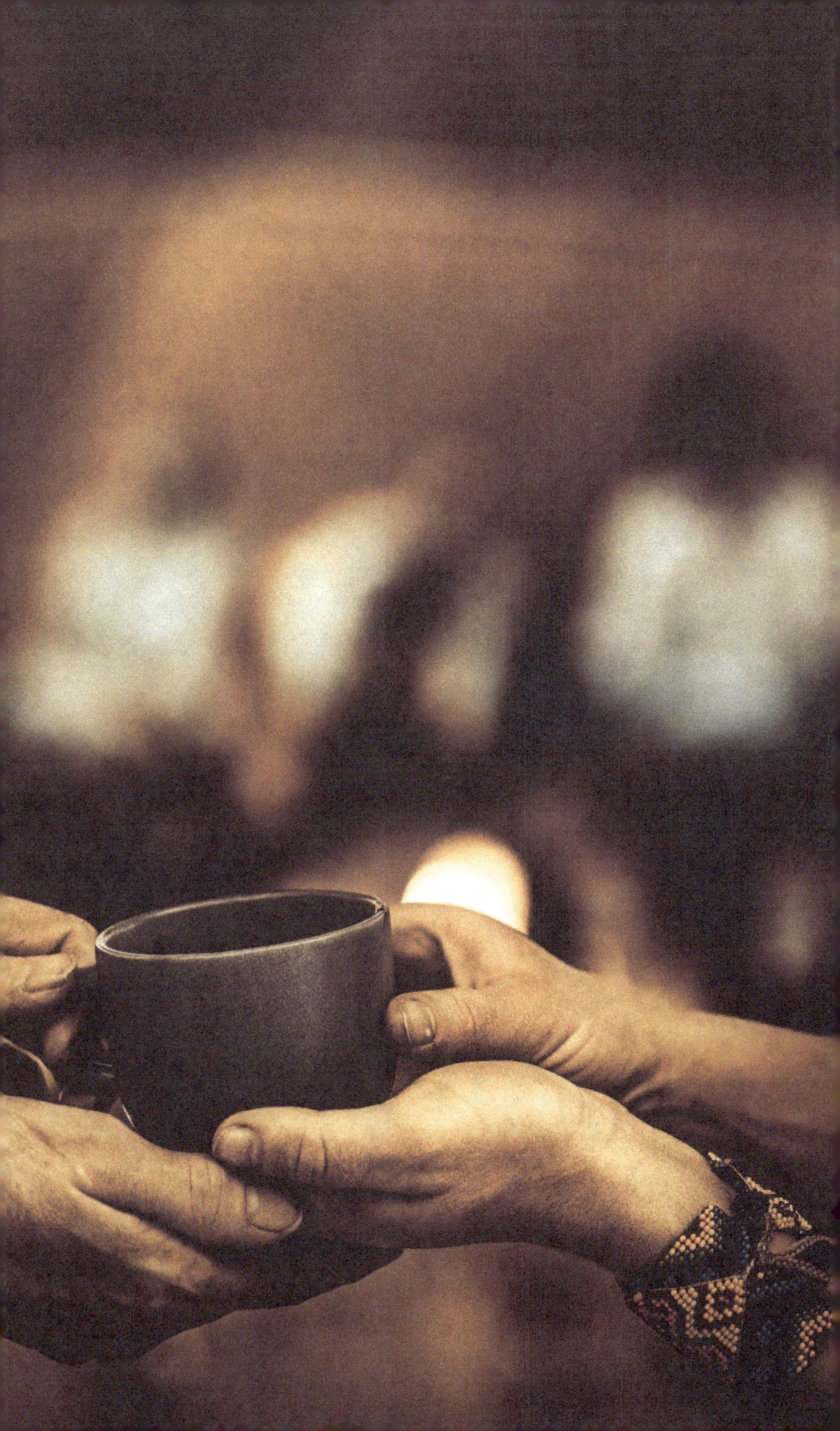

Chapter 4: The Cacao Celebration

As autumn painted the vineyard in shades of amber and gold,
Mia and Ethan found themselves embarking on a new journey,
one that celebrated their deepened connection to each other
and their connection to their community, their chosen family and
natural family.
Inspired by a friend's suggestion, they decided to host a cacao
ceremony, a tribute to their love and commitment.

The preparations transformed their beloved cottage grounds into
an enchanting scene.

Ethan, with a blend of practicality and creativity, crafted a
rustic firepit that became the heart of their outdoor sanctuary.
Nestled in a clearing, the firepit was a masterful construction of
local stone, each piece carefully chosen and placed by Ethan's
skilled hands. The stones, rugged and earth-toned, formed a
perfectly imperfect circle, their textures telling stories of the land.
In the centre, logs were artfully arranged, poised to ignite into a
mesmerising dance of flames that would reach up to the star-
studded sky.

Around this central feature, Ethan created a cosy amphitheatre
using hay bales, strategically placed to embrace the firepit.
Each bale was a seat of natural warmth, covered with layers
of blankets in rich, earthy hues, inviting guests to settle in and
enjoy the primal allure of the fire. The conscious and thoughtful
arrangement turned the space into a warm welcoming haven
under the open sky.

As night falls, the firepit will come alive with flickering flames,
casting a golden glow to illuminate the faces of friends and family
gathered around. The crackling of the fire will blend with the soft
rustle of the trees, creating a symphony of nature's music.

Mia transformed their gathering's entrance into a breathtaking
vision of autumn. She created an arch, embodying the season's
beauty and their deep love. More than a structure, it was

an enchanting portal, blending nature's magic with human connection.

Crafted from intertwined willow and birch branches, the arch radiated rustic charm, its natural curve forming an elegant frame. It was adorned with a vibrant array of backyard flowers and foliage, each piece carefully chosen to embody autumn. Plump, deep red dahlias and bright goldenrods added vivid splashes of colour, while sprigs of eucalyptus and strands of ivy infused the air with a tranquil fragrance and symbolised enduring love.

Hanging clusters of grapes paid homage to Ethan's vineyard work, complemented by whimsical pumpkins and gourds. Fairy lights woven through the arch bathed it in a soft, ethereal glow, creating a dreamlike atmosphere.

Guests walking under its canopy were wrapped in wonder, entering a realm where love was honoured and the everyday became magical.

The guests began to arrive - wrapped in scarves and smiles, and bearing arms full of delicious food to share - were greeted by this heavenly setup.
Each guest, an honoured friend or family member had a space in the circle, marked by blankets and trays that held beautiful, handmade pottery cups – a thoughtful gift from a friend and local artisan. The air was thick with anticipation and the sweet aroma of the earthy cacao wafted on the air.

The ceremony was led by Jenni, a long time friend of Ethans who Mia had become close to over the last few years, sharing tantric practices, exchanging gifts from their respective gardens and often losing track of time as the shared the ups and downs of life. Jenni was an experienced Circle Leader, whose gentle voice and soothing words guided them through the ritual.

Standing under the arch, Jenni opened the ceremony with a simple meditation, connecting the guests to each other and with Mother Nature.

Eternal Flames

She turned to the alter on the left - a heart-shaped arrangement using cacao beans, crystals and flowers from the garden to symbolise love and the heart-opening properties of cacao - and prepared the cacao. Gently blending the cacoa and water until it was rich, dark and fragrant.

Under a canopy of twinkling stars, they served the heart-opening cacao from an earthen pottery teapot, its surface etched with intricate designs that spoke of tradition and care.
Each pour of the rich, dark liquid into the waiting cups was a symbolic gesture of their nurturing love, an offering to their guests.

The aroma of the cacao, earthy and potent, filled the air. As the guests cradled their cups, the warmth of the drink seeped into their hands, radiating a sense of comfort and connection. The first sips were taken in thoughtful silence, a shared acknowledgment of the ceremony's significance.

One by one, the guests stepped forward, their eyes reflecting the fire's light, to bestow their blessings upon Mia and Ethan. Their words, heartfelt and sincere, wove a rich tapestry of goodwill, love and deep affection.
Some spoke of the couple's journey, others of the beauty of their union, each blessing adding to an atmosphere thick with emotion and a sense of sacredness.

Smiles, tears and gentle nods of agreement, each person present visibly moved by the ceremony's profound simplicity and the palpable love in the air.
The power of their collective goodwill, directed towards Mia and Ethan, created a moment of sublime connection, leaving an indelible imprint on everyone's heart.

Jenni gently drew the ceremony to a close, the atmosphere aglow with warmth and joy.
The guests, now a part of something magical, indulged in post-ritual snacks. Ethan's favorite wine vintages, products of his loving toil, flowed freely. The food, a cornucopia of homegrown delights, was a testament to the community's shared effort and love for Mia and Ethan.

The evening blossomed into a celebration of music and laughter. Fred who seemed to be born with a guitar in hand, initiated the singalong, his melodies harmonising with the chorus of voices. The songs, a blend of joy and nostalgia, echoed through the vineyard.

More than a ceremony, tonight was a manifestation of community, love, and the enriching experiences borne from sharing life's milestones. Their story, woven into the tapestry of their friends and family, continues to unfold.

Cacao Ceremony

This cacao ceremony is a beautiful blend of ritual, heartfelt sharing and community bonding, capturing the essence of Mia and Ethan's ceremony.
Includes variations for personalising for your requirements.

Total Duration: 60-90 minutes

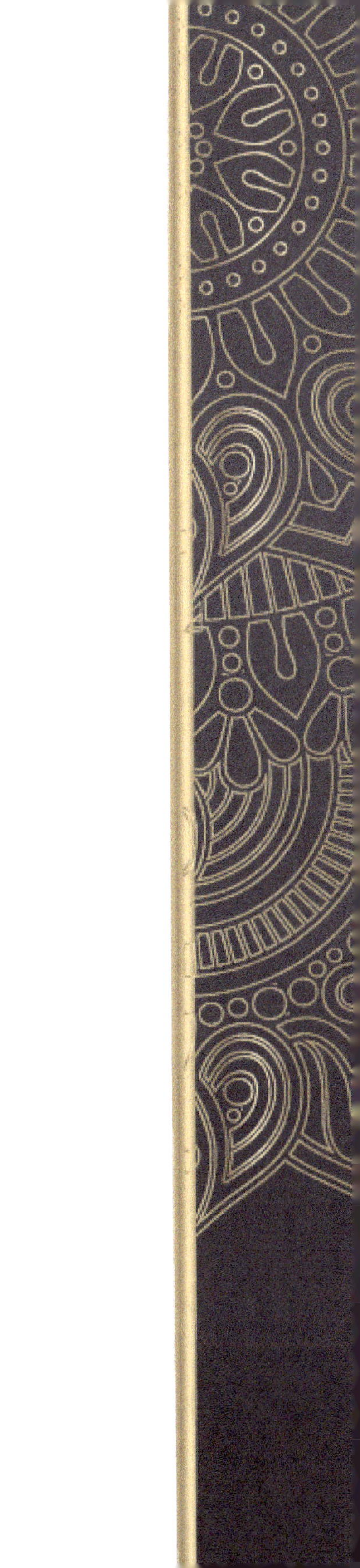

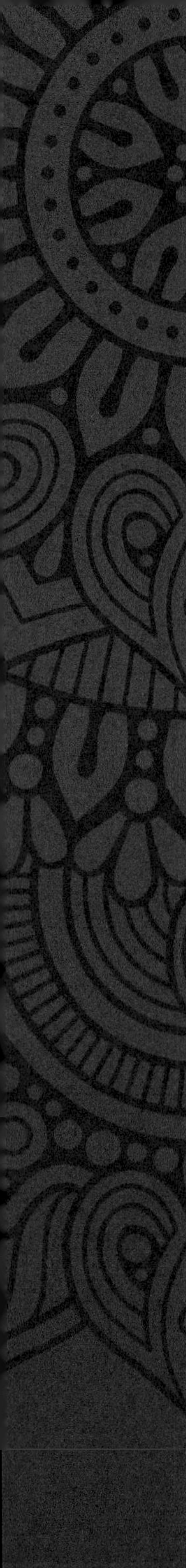

Preparation:

Setting the Space:
Choose a serene and comfortable location, preferably outdoors under the night sky.
Create a circular seating arrangement using cushions, ensuring everyone faces each other.
In the centre, set up a small table or altar adorned with natural elements like stones, crystals and flowers to symbolise the connection to Earth.
Light candles or lanterns around the space to create a warm, inviting glow.

The Cacao:
Prepare the cacao mixture beforehand using high-quality, ceremonial-grade cacao.
Gently heat it with water or milk, adding spices like cinnamon or chilli for warmth and flavour.

Ceremony Flow:

Welcoming the Guests:
As guests arrive, greet them with a warm, personal welcome, inviting them to take a seat in the circle.
Begin with a brief introduction about the significance of the cacao ceremony, focusing on themes of love, connection, and heart-opening.

Opening the Circle:
Start by creating a sacred space. Invite everyone to close their eyes and take deep, grounding breaths.
Lead a short meditation focusing on heart-opening and connection to the present moment.

Serving the Cacao:
option 1 -
Hosts begin serving the cacao, slowly pour the warm liquid into each guest's cup, moving around the circle.
option 2 -
Host or Circle Leader fills a cup and passes it on the next person who passes on until all guests have a cup.

Encourage guests to hold their cups with both hands, feeling the warmth, and to set a personal intention before the first sip.

Sharing and Blessings:
Once everyone has their cacao, open the floor for sharing. This can be in the form of blessings like for Mia and Ethan if it is for a personal ceremony, or for the more usual ceremony invite personal reflections, or expressions relevant to the overal theme based on each persons experience.
Create a supportive atmosphere where each person feels heard and valued. Allow each person shares, allow them to speak freely for 1 -3 minutes without interupting or asking questions. When the time is complete, ring a little bell as a signal to move to the next guest.

Heartfelt Expressions:
Incorporate elements of music, poetry, or gentle movement to allow guests to express themselves and engage with the ceremony on a deeper level.
This can be an open space for guests to share a song, a dance, or a piece of poetry that resonates with the theme.

Closing the Circle:
Conclude the ceremony by bringing everyone's focus back to the circle.
Offer thanks and reflections on the blessings and shares.
End with a group embrace or a collective deep breath, symbolising unity and shared experience.

Post-Ceremony Gathering:
Invite guests to linger, enjoy light refreshments and conversations. This allows for the deepening of connections and the formation of new friendships.

Considerations:
Ensure the ceremony is inclusive and respectful of all participants.
Be mindful of the amount of cacao served, as it can be potent.
The ceremony should be a safe space for emotional expression and sharing.

5: New Horizons
Mia's Journey of Discovery

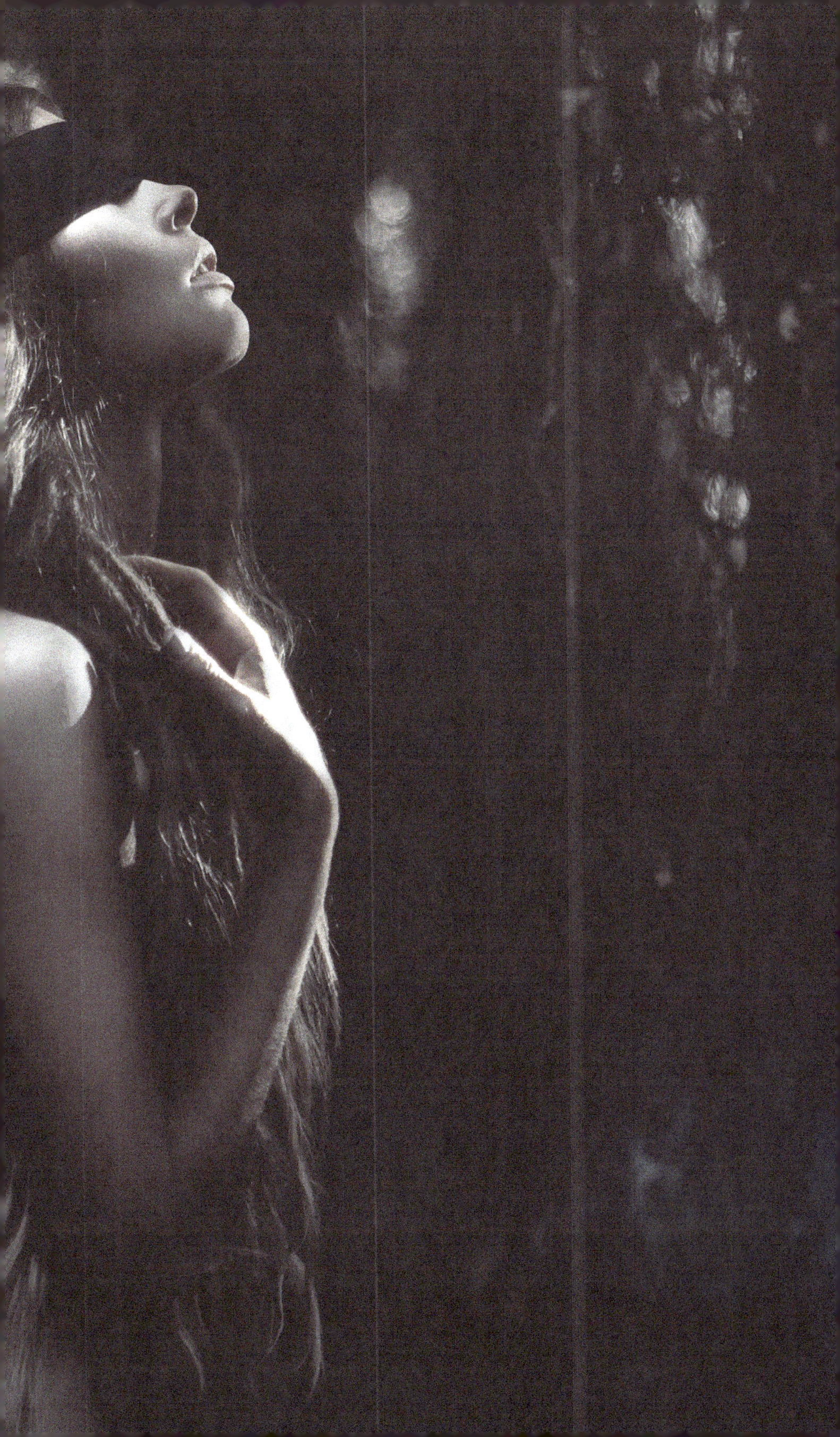

Chapter 5: New Horizons
Mia's Journey of Discovery

In the evolving landscape of their lives, Mia and Ethan had nurtured a relationship that blossomed with deep spiritual connections and the exploration of uncharted territories.

Their commitment to sustainable living, tantric practices, and open relationships had not only strengthened their bond but also opened their hearts to others who shared similar values. It was in this nurturing environment that Mia found herself inexplicably drawn to Elara, a woman whose essence resonated deeply with her own.

Elara, a frequent visitor to their cottage, was a soul connected intimately with nature, possessing a profound grasp of tantric principles. Her presence brought a rejuvenating energy and new perspectives to Mia and Ethan's world.
With Elara, Mia felt a bond that transcended friendship, stirring a curiosity and desire to explore this connection further.

Recognizing the potential depth of their growing bond, Mia and Elara decided to embark on a discovery ritual, a practice deeply rooted in tantra, to explore and understand the nuances of their connection.

As the evening unfolded, the cottage transformed into a sanctuary of discovery. Candles cast a soft, inviting glow and the air was fragrant with the scent of jasmine.
In the living room, Mia and Elara set the stage for their ritual, arranging cushions in a circle around a small altar adorned with symbols reflecting their intentions.

 Mia and Elara sat facing each other, the candlelight flickering in their eyes. Mia spoke first, her voice a mix of excitement and vulnerability. "I wish to explore this new path with you, to understand your spirit, and to honour our journey together," she said.
Elara responded with equal sincerity, expressing her desire to deepen their bond and share in the energy of their growing connection.

In the circle's embrace, they began with synchronized breathing, inhaling and exhaling in unison. This shared rhythm brought them into a harmonious alignment, bridging their energies and fostering a sense of unity.

The ritual deepened as they placed their hands over each other's heart chakras, their left hands remaining on their own. With eyes closed, they visualized a vibrant flow of energy between their hearts, a dynamic exchange that was both nurturing and empowering.

The room then filled with a silent, communicative dance of touch. They explored each other's hands, arms, and shoulders with gentle curiosity, each touch a word in their unspoken dialogue.

This was a journey of understanding and connection, exploring the physical and energetic presence of one another.

Reconnecting eye to eye, they shared affirmations, their words weaving a tapestry of empowerment and acceptance. They acknowledged the beauty of their individual journeys and the potential richness of their combined paths.

As the ritual drew to a close, they shared reflections on their experience, each feeling enriched and connected. They concluded with a heartfelt embrace, a symbol of their mutual respect and the deep connection they had fostered.

In the waning candlelight, Mia felt a profound sense of gratitude and wonder. The ritual with Elara had opened a new horizon in her journey, promising a deeper exploration and discovery. In her heart, she knew this was just the beginning of a beautiful journey, a dance of souls that would add new dimensions to her life and enrich the journey she shared with Ethan.

Tantric Discovery Ritual

This ritual is designed for two people who wish to deepen their connection and explore each other's energies on an intermediate level. It's a journey of mutual discovery, fostering intimacy, understanding, and a deeper spiritual bond.

Total Duration: 45-60 minutes

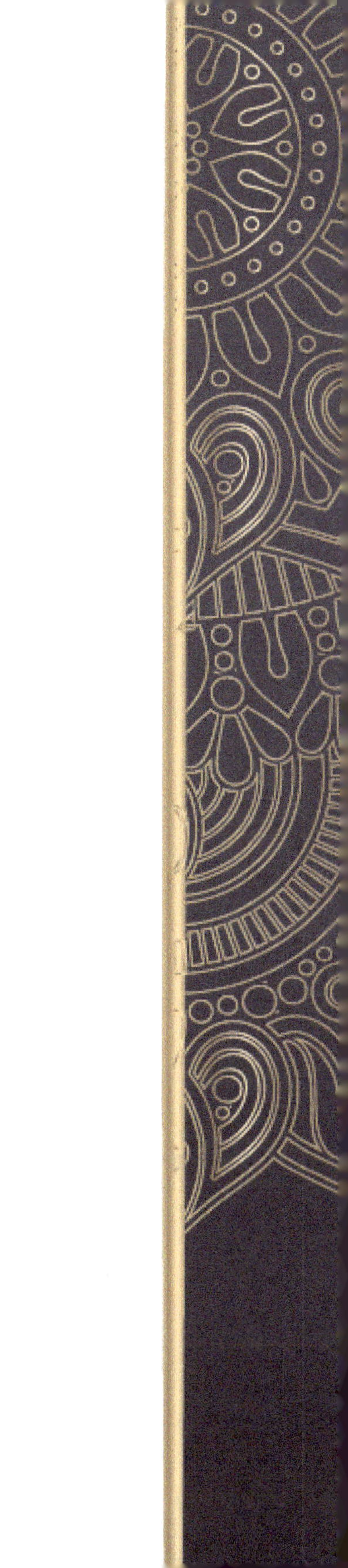

Preparation:
Set up a quiet, comfortable space free from distractions.
Place cushions or mats for sitting and lying down.
Light candles to create a soft, inviting glow and play gentle,
ambient music to enhance the atmosphere.

Grounding and Centering (5 minutes):
Joint Breathing: Sit facing each other with eyes closed
and begin by synchronizing your breathing. Inhale and
exhale deeply together, establishing a shared rhythm and
connection.

Four Pillars of Connection (20 minutes):
Eye Gazing (5 minutes): Open your eyes and engage in
eye gazing. Maintain a soft, gentle gaze, connecting non-
verbally. This practice fosters a deep sense of presence and
connection.

Synchronized Heartbeat (5 minutes):
Place your right hand on your partner's heart and your left
hand over your own heart. Feel each other's heartbeat and
try to synchronize your breathing with it.

Energy Sensing (5 minutes):
Hover your hands slightly above your partner's body without
touching, moving your hands along their energy field. Feel
the warmth and energy radiating from their body.

Harmonious Mantra Chanting (5 minutes):
Together chant a simple mantra like "Om" or "So Hum."
Focus on the vibration and harmony of your voices uniting.

Mindful Touch Exploration (10 minutes):
Gentle Caress: Take turns to gently explore each other's
arms, hands, and shoulders with respectful touch,
communicating warmth and affection. Remain attuned to
each other's reactions and comfort levels.

Shared Breath and Energy Flow (10 minutes):
Harmonized Breathing: Sit in the Yab-Yum position (one person sitting on the other's lap, facing each other) or side by side. Breathe in unison, imagining a shared flow of energy circulating between your bodies.

Visualizing Connection: Visualize a stream of light or energy connecting your heart chakras, deepening the sense of unity and empathy.

Affirmations and Intentions (5 minutes):
Exchange of Words: Share affirmations or intentions with each other. Speak words of appreciation, understanding, or shared goals for your journey together.

Closing the Ritual:
Gratitude and Acknowledgment: Conclude the ritual by expressing gratitude for the experience and for each other's presence and openness.

Gentle Transition: Slowly transition out of the ritual space, maintaining a sense of calm and connection.

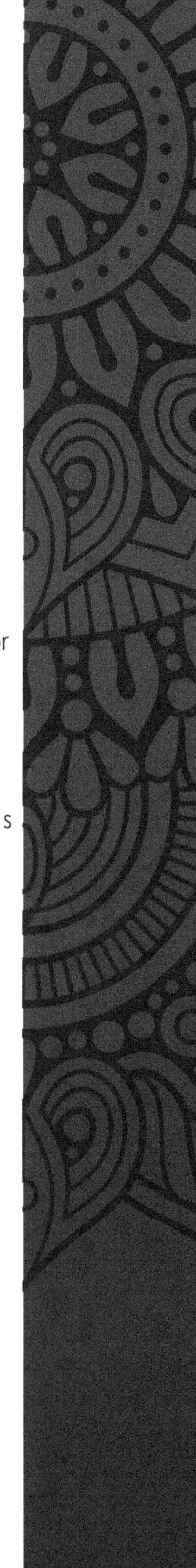

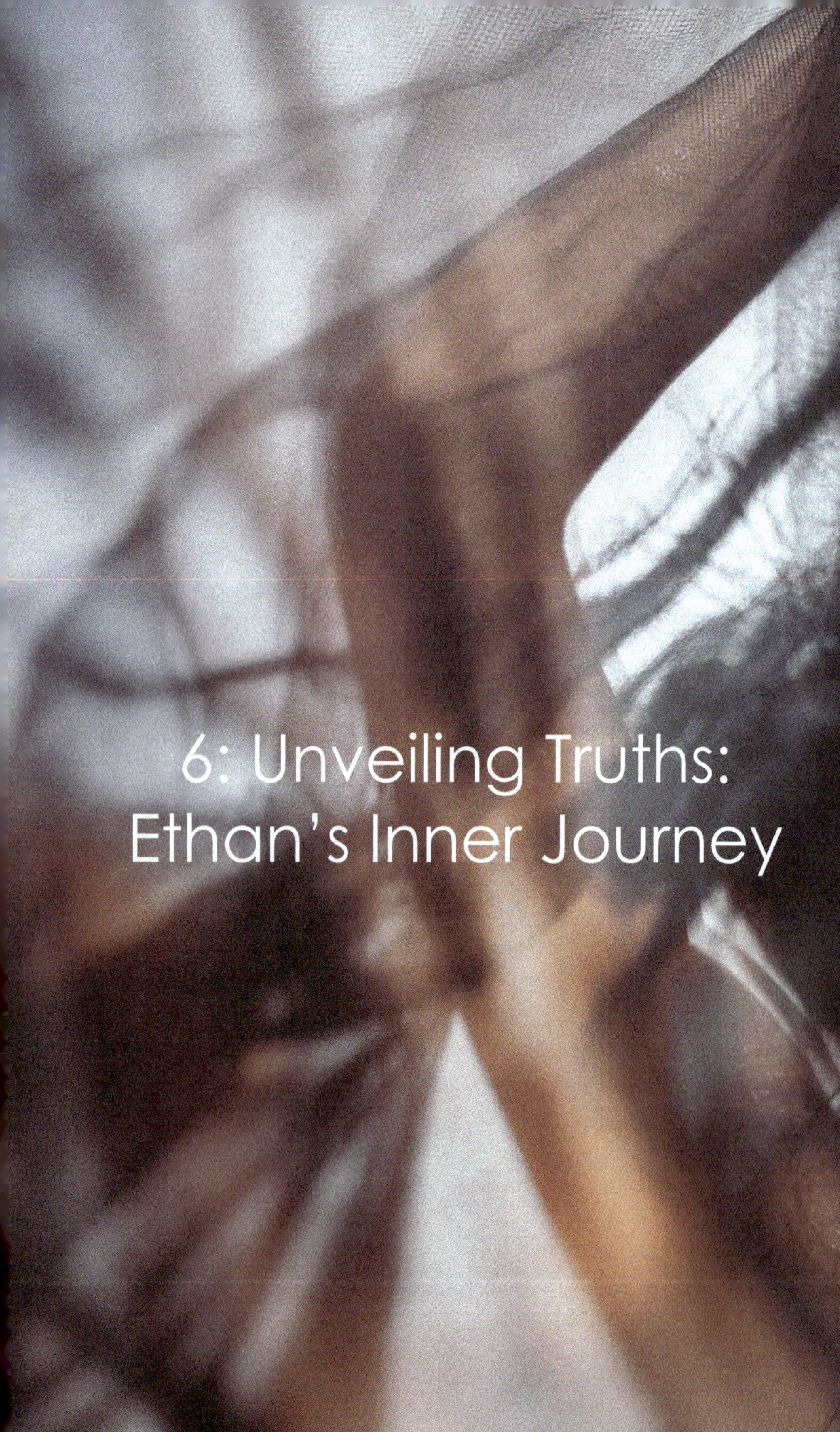
6: Unveiling Truths:
Ethan's Inner Journey

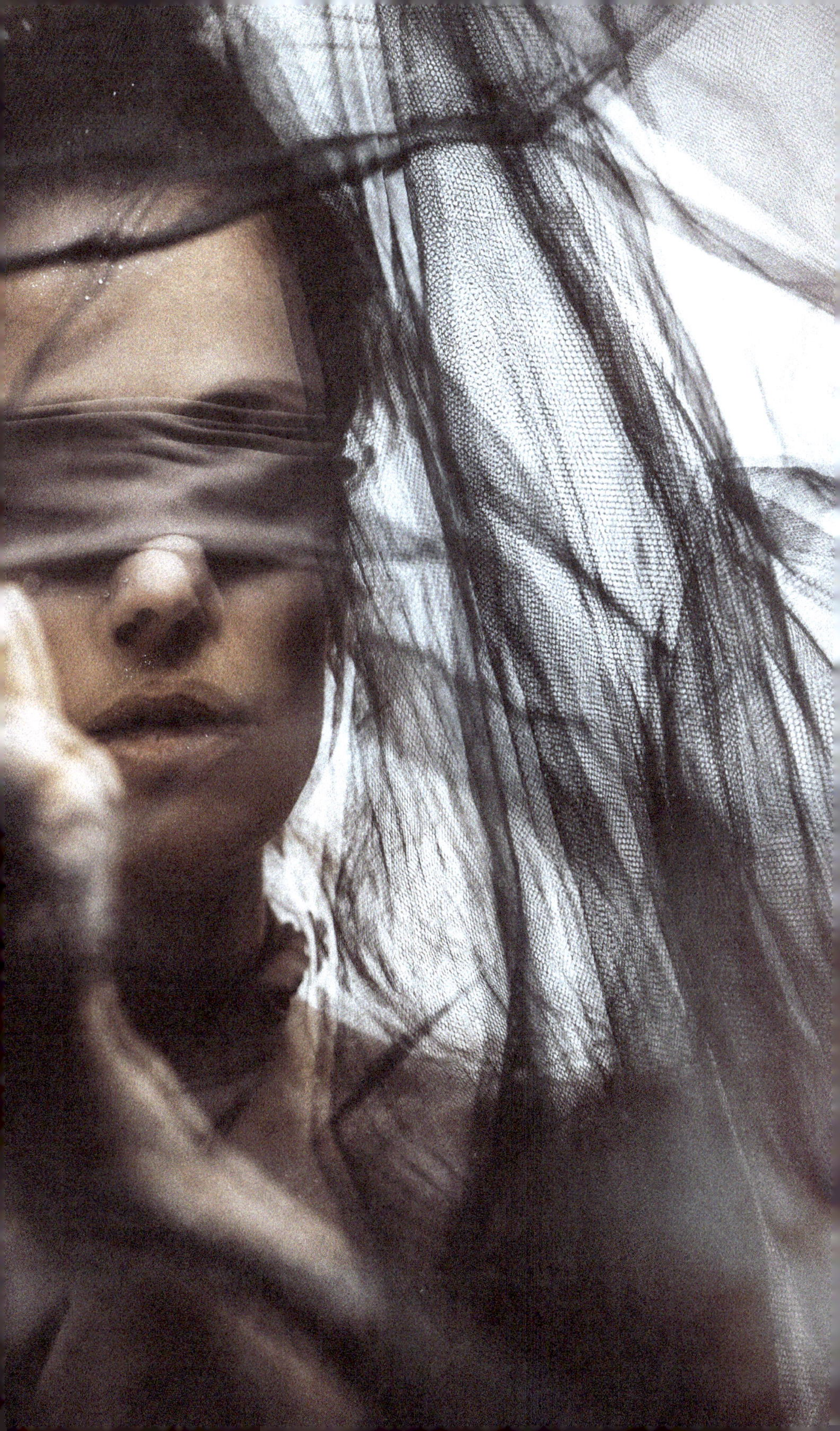

Chapter 6: Unveiling Truths: Ethan's Inner Journey

In the evolving tapestry of their relationship, Mia and Ethan had embraced a life of openness, welcoming others who shared their values of sustainable living and tantric practices.

This journey into an open, multi-partner relationship had brought many enriching experiences, but it also presented its unique set of challenges. For Ethan, Mia's recent relationship with another man, Lucas, stirred a tumult of emotions that he hadn't anticipated.

Ethan, always a proponent of open-mindedness and exploration, found himself grappling with feelings of insecurity and jealousy. These feelings were unfamiliar in their shared journey, and they cast a shadow of doubt on the way Ethan understood their relationship. He knew that these emotions needed to be addressed, not just for his peace but for the integrity of his and Mia's bond.

Realising the need for open communication, Ethan proposed a truth-telling ritual, a sacred space where he could share his fears with Mia, and they could reaffirm their connection.

On the night of the ritual, they created a circle of trust in their living room, surrounded by the soothing presence of candles and the comforting aroma of sandalwood. They sat facing each other, their eyes reflecting the seriousness and the love that underpinned their relationship.

Ethan began by setting the intention for their ritual.
"This space is for honesty, for sharing our deepest truths without fear or judgment," he declared.
Mia nodded, her eyes conveying her support and willingness to listen.

Together, they engaged in deep breathing exercises, a practice to help Ethan release tension and prepare his heart for sharing. With each breath, Ethan felt his apprehensions lessen, making way for clarity and vulnerability.

Ethan took the lead, sharing his feelings about Mia's relationship with Lucas. "I feel a sense of loss," he admitted, "as though I'm not enough, or that our bond might be overshadowed."
Mia listened, her presence a comforting anchor as Ethan navigated through his mix of emotions.

Mia, practicing active listening, acknowledged Ethan's feelings without interruption, letting him know that his emotions were valid and heard.

"Your feelings matter," she assured him, her voice gentle but firm.

Mia then shared her perspective, reinforcing her love and commitment to Ethan. "Our journey is unique, and no other relationship can diminish what we have," she said.
They discussed ways to ensure that their primary bond remained strong and secure, even as they explored connections with others.

To conclude the ritual, they engaged in a reconnection exercise, holding hands and gazing into each other's eyes, reaffirming their primary partnership.

They ended with a deep embrace, a physical manifestation of their enduring bond and renewed understanding.

As the ritual came to a close, Ethan felt a weight lift from his shoulders. The act of sharing his fears and hearing Mia's reaffirmation had rekindled a sense of security and trust.

He realised that the path they had chosen was not without its complexities, but it was their shared honesty and love that would guide them through any challenge.

Mia and Ethan's journey together was a continuous exploration of love, trust, and understanding. This truth-telling ritual had not only allowed Ethan to confront and share his vulnerabilities but had also strengthened the foundation of their ever-evolving relationship.

Truth Telling Ritual

This ritual is designed to deepen the connection between partners through honest communication and shared vulnerability. It combines elements of tantric practices with the power of truth-telling to foster intimacy and understanding.

Total Duration: 45-60 minutes

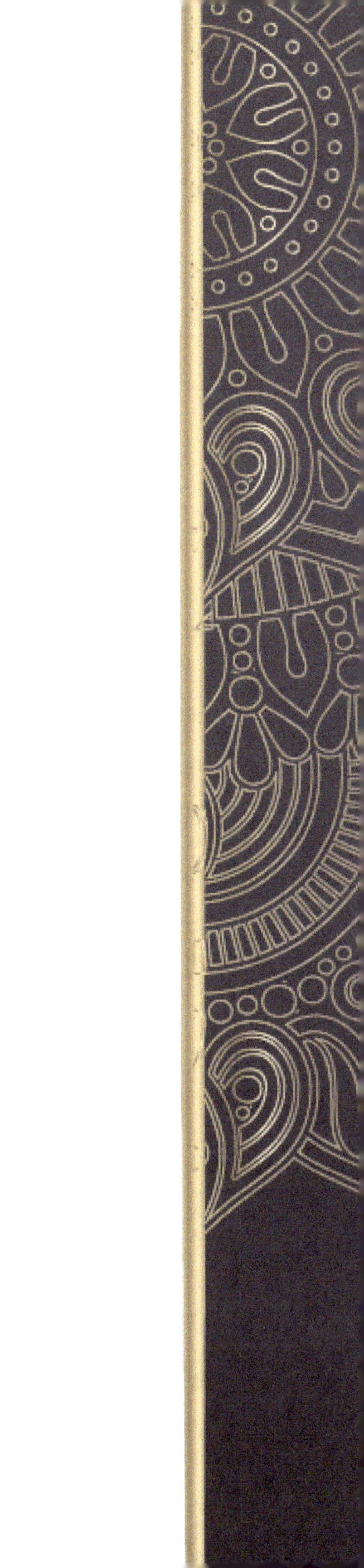

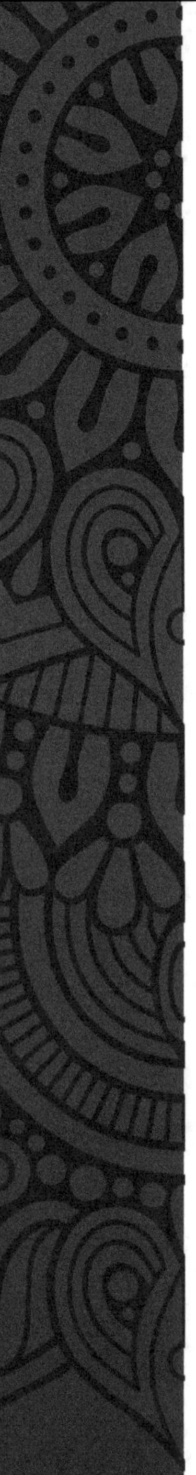

Preparation:
Create a Comfortable Space: Choose a quiet, private space where you won't be disturbed. Sit facing each other on cushions or chairs at a comfortable distance.

Set the Ambiance: Dim the lights or light candles to create a serene atmosphere. Consider playing soft, ambient music in the background.

Grounding and Centring (2 minutes):
Synchronized Breathing: Begin by closing your eyes and taking deep, synchronised breaths. Inhale and exhale together to create a rhythm, focusing on the sound and feel of your breath.

Establishing a Safe Space (2 minutes):
Setting Intentions: Open your eyes and take turns to express your intention for the ritual. This could be to speak and receive truth with love, to understand each other better, or to deepen your connection.

Guided Visualisation (3 minutes):
Creating a Connection: Still holding eye contact, visualize a beam of light connecting your hearts. This light represents the love and trust between you, growing stronger with each breath.

Truth-Telling Exercise (5 minutes):
Sharing Truths: Take turns sharing something you feel, need, or have been hesitant to express. Speak honestly but with kindness. The partner listening should do so without interrupting, offering their full attention.

Active Listening: When one partner speaks, the other should practice active listening — a key component of tantric communication. This means listening with empathy, without planning a response or judgment.

Affirmation and Acknowledgment (2 minutes):
Acknowledging Each Other: After both partners have shared, acknowledge what you've heard with simple statements like "I hear you" or "Thank you for sharing that with me." This helps validate each other's feelings and experiences.

Reconnection and Gratitude (3 minutes):
Heart-Centred Gratitude: Place your hand on your heart and one hand on your partner's heart. Share one thing you appreciate about each other.

Closing the Ritual:
Conclude the ritual with a hug or a loving gesture, reaffirming your connection and gratitude for the shared experience.

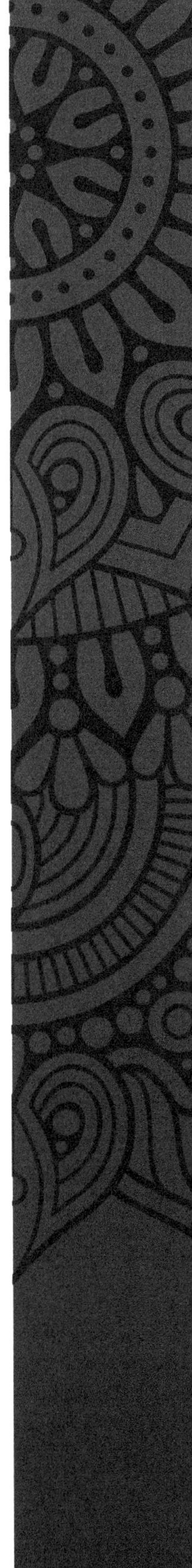

7: Expanding Horizons: Ethan and Lucas's Exploration

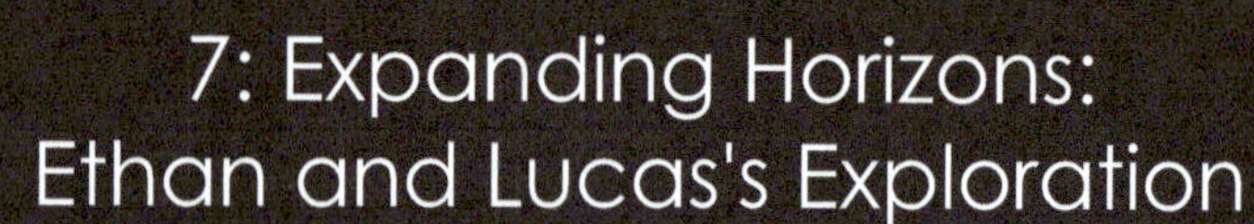

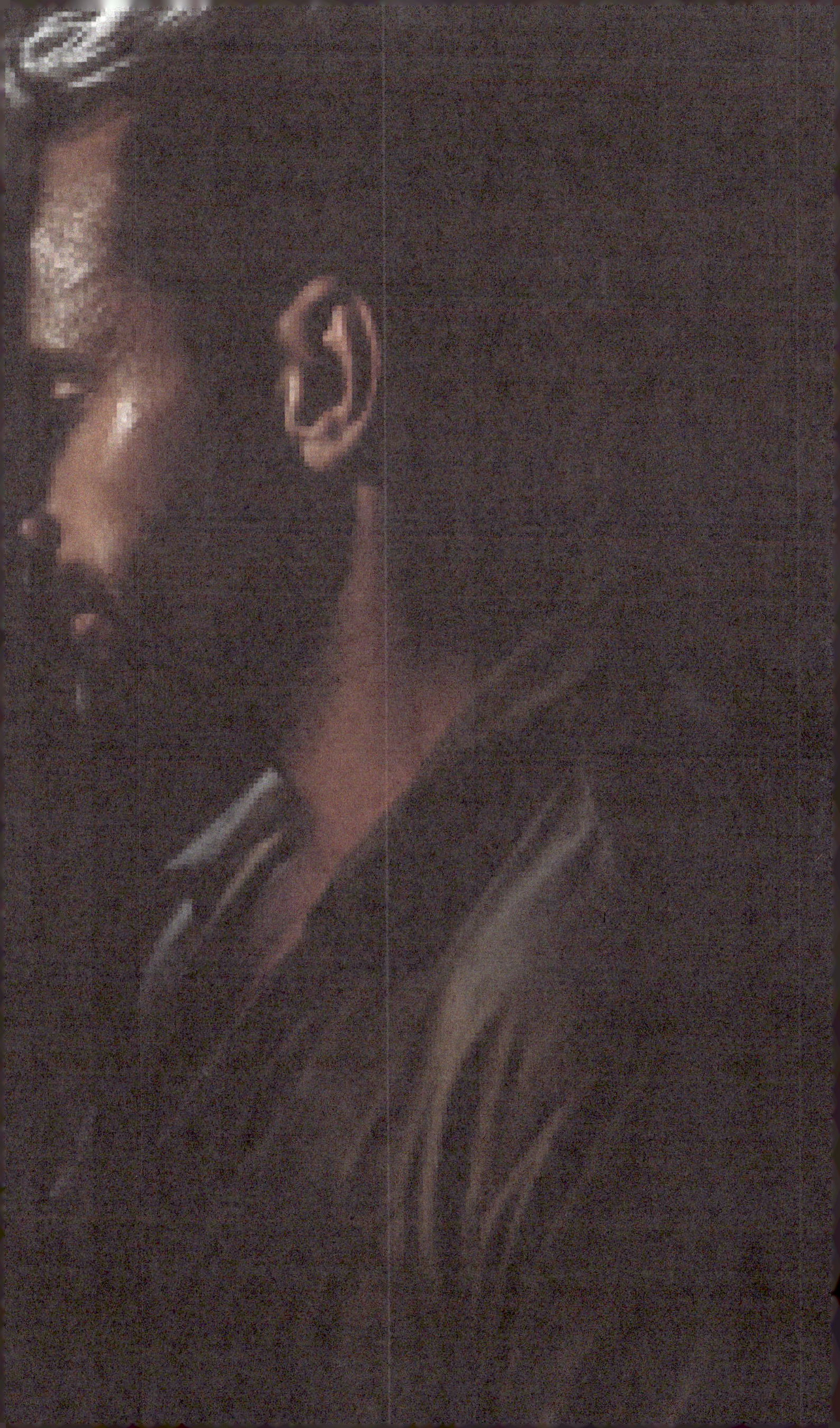

Chapter 7: Expanding Horizons: Ethan and Lucas's Exploration

In the heart of their evolving relationship, Mia and Ethan's journey had always been one of open exploration and profound honesty. Their bond, rooted in the principles of tantra and a deep, spiritual connection, had gracefully withstood the tests of time and change.
It was within this nurturing environment that Ethan found himself at the threshold of a new and unexpected path with Lucas, Mia's partner.

Ethan, always guided by a spirit of openness and self-discovery, had come to a profound realisation during their truth-telling ritual. He confessed to Mia and Lucas a long-held curiosity about the experience of intimacy with another man.

This revelation, far from creating a rift, opened a door to deeper understanding and exploration. Lucas, who also harboured a bi-curiosity, resonated with Ethan's feelings and together they agreed to explore this newfound connection.

The journey that Ethan and Lucas embarked upon was cautious yet exhilarating. Their initial explorations were tender and hesitant, each man navigating the uncharted waters of their emotions and desires.
Their first kiss, a hesitant yet electric meeting of lips was a moment of profound vulnerability and discovery. They delved deeper, exploring gentle embraces, the warmth of each other's presence, discovering strength and courage.
They found in each other an unexpected source of comfort and understanding.

Mia, witnessing the unfolding of this new connection between Ethan and Lucas, felt an overwhelming sense of joy and fulfillment. She saw the men in her life exploring deeper parts of themselves, and it only deepened her love and respect for them.
Her support and enthusiasm were unwavering, a testament to the strength and openness of their relationship.

Over the following months, the intimate dynamics of Mia and

Ethan's open relationship evolved into a flexible arrangement that included Lucas and Elara.

They found themselves navigating a complex web of relationships, sometimes as couples, threesomes, or all together. This fluidity of connections presented its unique set of challenges, as four individuals with different needs, schedules and emotional attachments tried to harmonise their lives.

The journey was not without its hurdles. Balancing time, attention and emotional energy among four people plus occasional other visitors into the arrangement required a level of communication and honesty that was sometimes daunting.
Jealousies and insecurities surfaced, challenging each individual to confront their fears and embrace vulnerability.

Through these challenges, they relied heavily on their practice of tantra and their commitment to truthfulness. They held regular rituals, similar to the one that had brought Ethan and Lucas together, allowing each person to express their feelings, fears, and desires openly. These rituals became sacred spaces of healing, understanding, and reconnection.

As the years passed, the four of them wove a rich and complex tapestry of relationships. Their bond, nourished by honesty and a deep understanding of each other's needs, grew stronger and more resilient.
They found joy in the flexibility of their arrangement, celebrating each other's individuality while maintaining a harmonious balance.

This experience was a testament to the power of love, communication and openness. In embracing their truths and exploring the depths of their connections, Mia, Ethan, Lucas, and Elara discovered a profound sense of fulfillment and happiness.

They had created a unique and beautiful harmony, a relationship that was as unconventional as it was deeply satisfying.

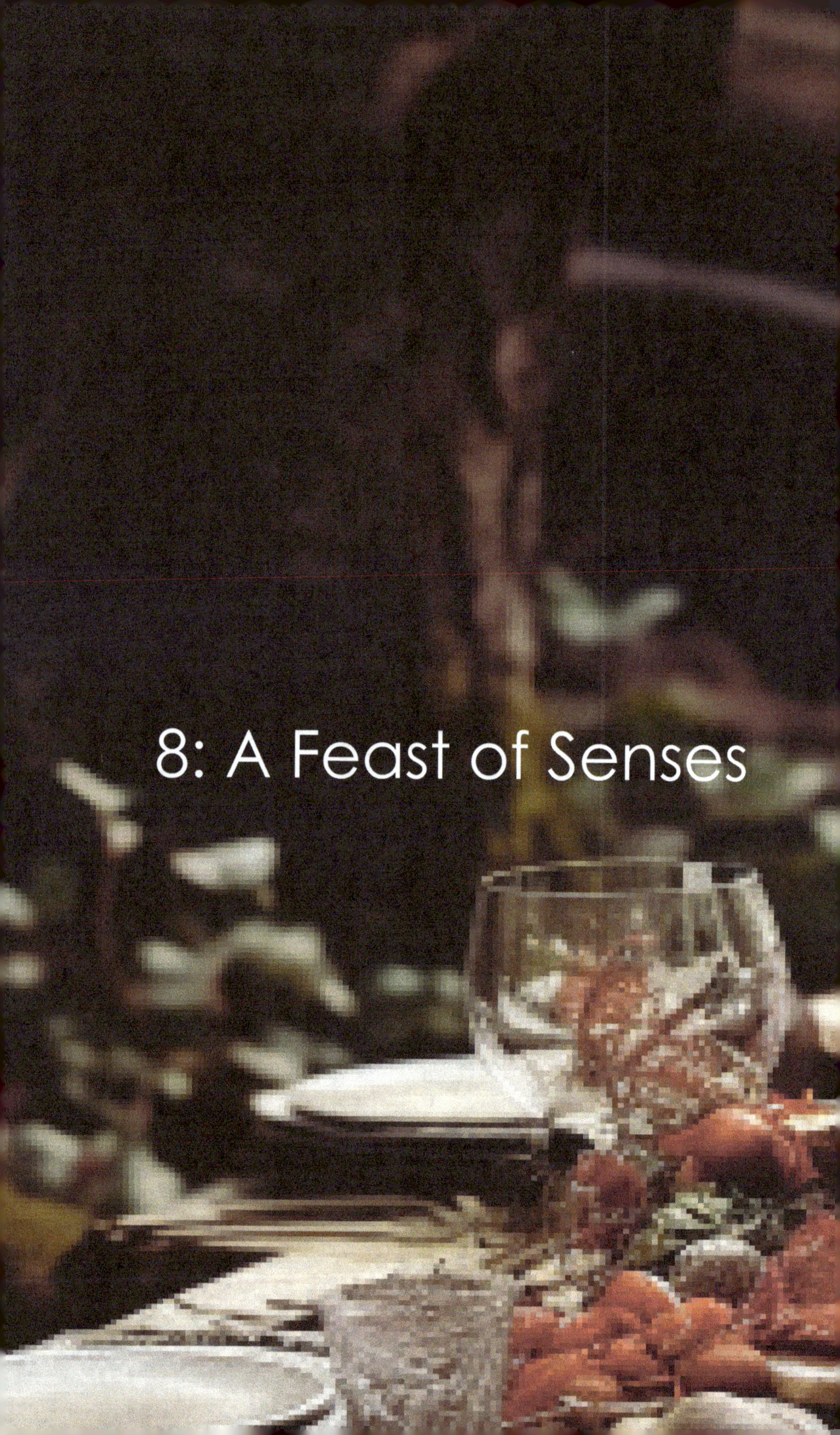
8: A Feast of Senses

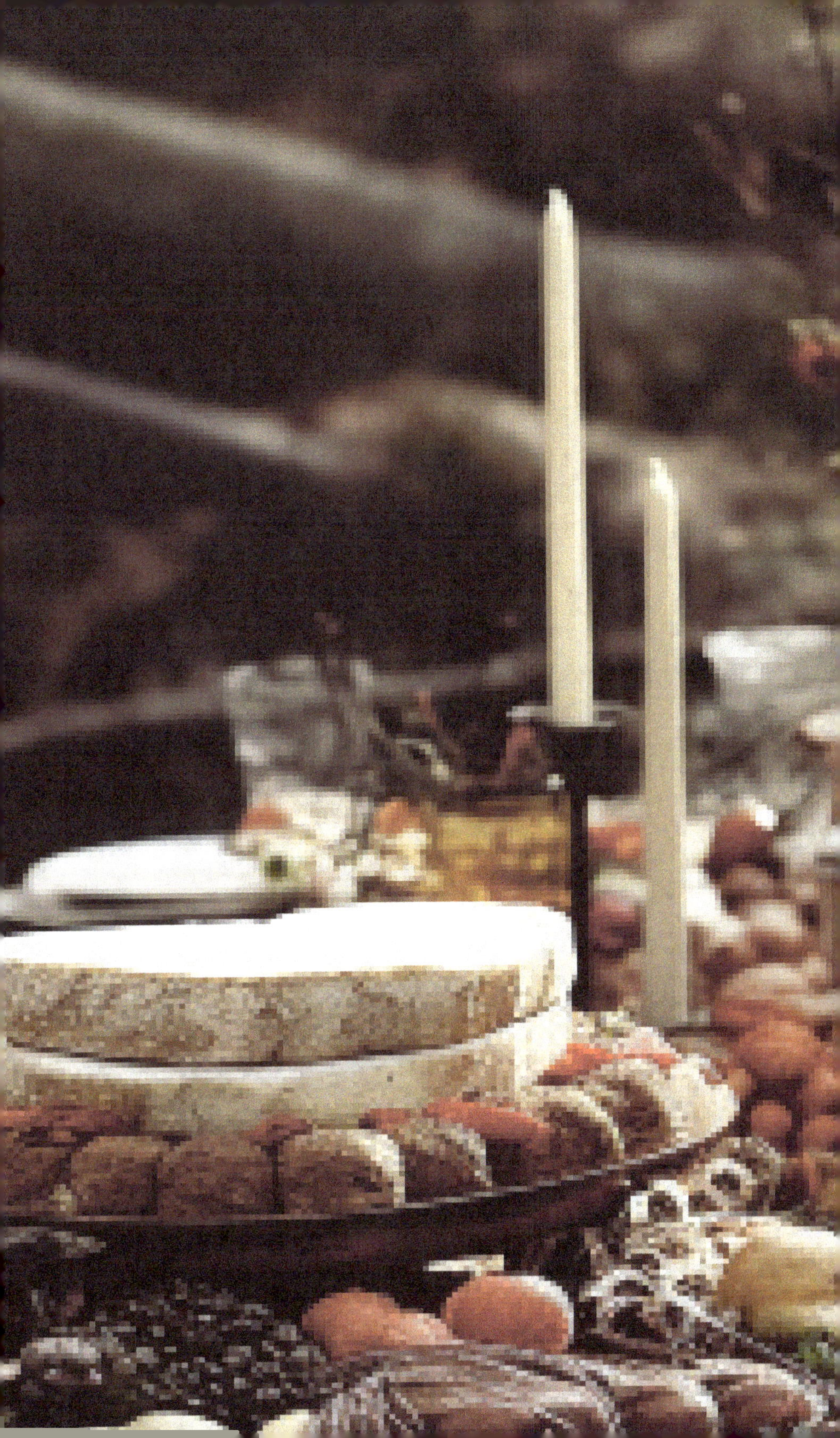

Chapter 8: A Feast of Senses and Souls

The journey of Mia and Ethan had evolved beautifully over the years, their bond deepening into a wellspring of spiritual and emotional intimacy.
Their cottage, nestled amidst the verdant vineyards of the Mornington Peninsula, had become a sanctuary not just for them, but also for a close-knit circle of friends who shared their values of sustainable living, open relationships, and a passion for tantric practices.

Tonight the cottage was alive with soft music, laughter and the rich aromas of a feast being prepared.
They were hosting a dinner party, but not just any dinner - it was to be an evening where food and tantra intertwined, celebrating their shared journey in a community of like-minded souls.

As the guests arrived, each bringing a dish crafted with love and care, the cottage hummed with a warm, inviting energy.
Mia, her hair tied back and her eyes sparkling with excitement, greeted each friend with a heartfelt hug.
Ethan, his presence calm and welcoming, ushered everyone into the heart of their home.

The dining area had been transformed. A large, low table lay in the center, surrounded by plush cushions. The table was adorned with an array of dishes - vibrant, fragrant and inviting. It was a tapestry of colours and scents, each dish telling a story of the hands that had crafted it.

Once everyone had settled, Mia and Ethan led the group in setting their intentions for the evening. Voices mingled in the candlelit room, each person sharing their hopes and thoughts, weaving a collective spirit of connection and exploration.

The ritual began with the mindful eating practice. Laughter and soft murmurs filled the air as each guest took turns choosing food for another, creating an intricate dance of giving and receiving.

Mia watched with a gentle smile as a friend offered her a slice of ripe fig, its sweetness bursting on her tongue, a symphony of flavour.

Ethan, in turn, selected a piece of artisanal cheese for a friend, his movements deliberate and full of care. As they ate, the room was enveloped in a shared reverence for the sensory experience, for the act of nourishment, and for the bonds being deepened with every bite.

As the evening unfolded, the guests shared their experiences. Tales of texture, aroma, and taste mingled with deeper reflections on trust, intimacy, and the joy of communal bonding. Each story added a layer to the rich tapestry of the night, a celebration of the senses and of the soul.

In the warmth of their cottage, surrounded by friends who had become family, Mia and Ethan felt a profound sense of gratitude. Their journey together had brought them here, to this moment of shared joy and spiritual communion, a testament to the paths they had chosen and the bonds they had nurtured.

As the night drew to a close, the group gathered for a final moment of reflection. Hands joined in a circle, hearts beating in unison, they took a moment to acknowledge the beauty of their connection, the magic of their shared journey.

In the flickering candlelight, Mia and Ethan exchanged a look of deep understanding and love. This evening was more than a dinner party; it was a celebration of their life together, of the open, multi-partner relationships that had enriched their world, and of the spiritual journey that continued to unfold in the heart of their little cottage.

As the guests departed, the cottage settled back into its usual quietude, but the echoes of laughter and heartfelt conversations lingered in the air.

Mia and Ethan, hand in hand, looked at each other, knowing that their journey was far from over, but for now, they reveled in the joy of this perfect moment in time.

Tantric Feast

This practice can be a beautiful way to connect, explore senses, and enhance the feeling of community and intimacy among friends or couples.
Approach the ritual with respect, openness and an intention to experience deeper connection and presence.

Total Duration: as long as it takes

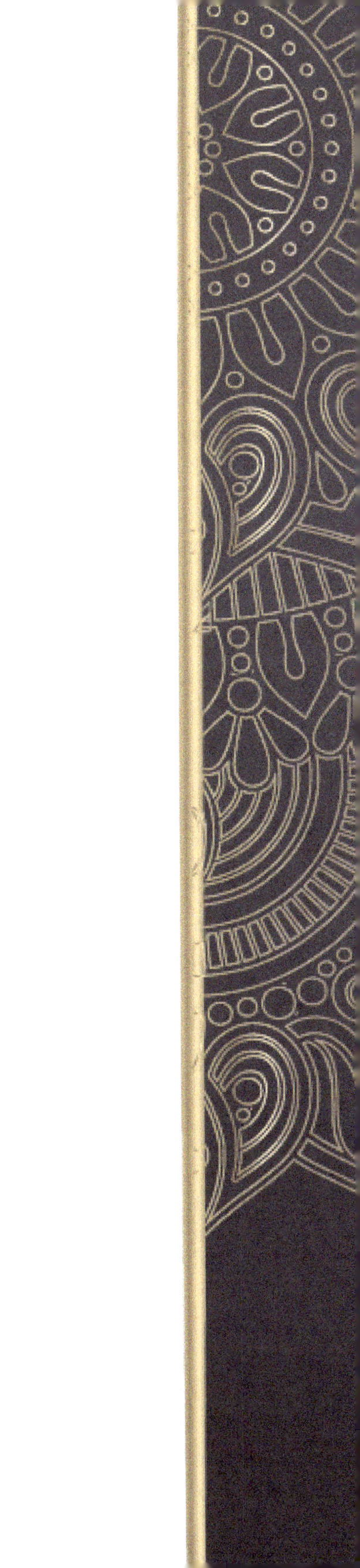

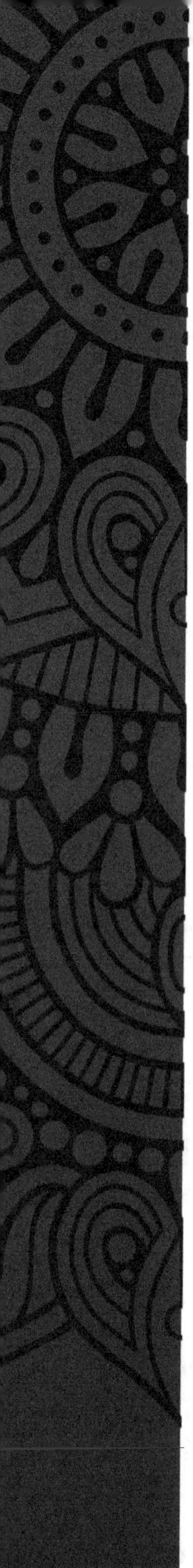

Preparation:

Create a comfortable and serene space. Place cushions or mats in a circle, ensuring everyone can see and easily interact with each other.

Choose a variety of foods that engage different senses: textures (smooth, crunchy), temperatures (warm, cool), and tastes (sweet, sour, salty, bitter, umami).
Include fruits, chocolates, nuts, cheese, and perhaps some exotic or unusual items.
Present the food beautifully on a central platter/s, accessible to all participants.

Setting the Intention (5 minutes):

Sit in the circle, close your eyes, and take a few deep breaths to centre yourselves.
One by one, share your intention for the practice. This could be to deepen connections, explore the senses, or simply to enjoy a shared experience.

Mindful Eating (15-20 minutes):

Begin the mindful eating practice. One person starts by choosing a piece of food for the person on their left, placing it on their plate or hand without verbal communication.

Before eating, each person takes a moment to observe the food, noticing its colour, texture and aroma.
Slowly taste the food, focusing on the sensations, flavours, and experience. Chew mindfully and savour each bite.

Continue the process in a clockwise direction, with each person selecting food for the next, allowing for a moment of connection as they offer the food.

Sharing the Experience (5-10 minutes):

After everyone has tasted a few items, take turns sharing your experiences. Discuss the sensations, emotions, and thoughts that arose during the mindful eating.
Reflect on the act of being fed by another and feeding

another, exploring themes of trust, nurturing, and connection.

Closing the Practice (5 minutes):
Conclude the practice by expressing gratitude for the food, the company, and the shared experience.
Sit in a moment of silent reflection or a group embrace, acknowledging the unique connection created through this practice.

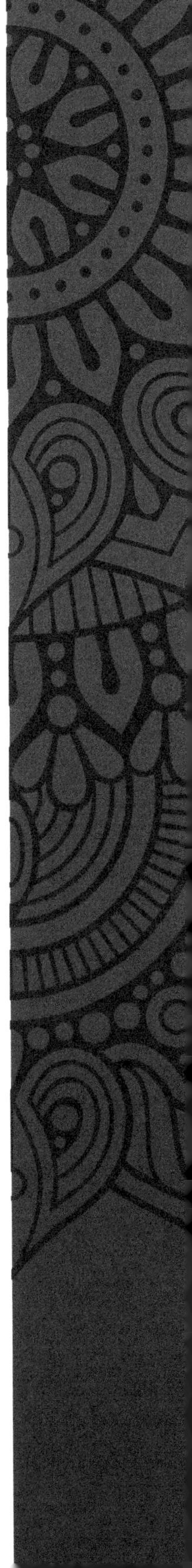

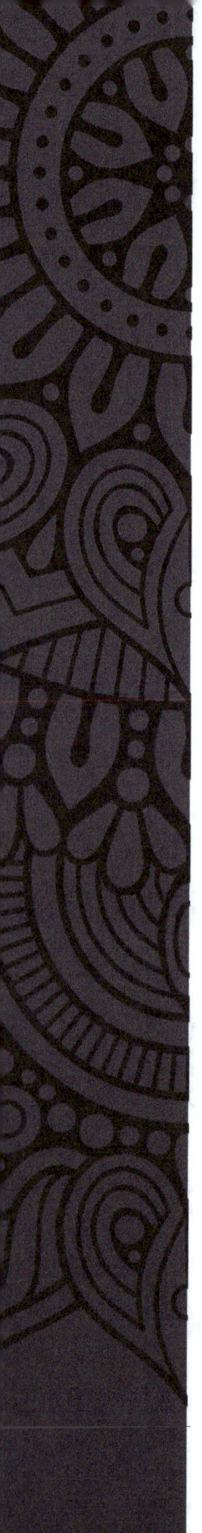

Tantric Feast Menu

Appetisers:

Herb-Infused Goat Cheese Crostini: Fresh herbs from the garden, combined with creamy goat cheese on toasted artisanal bread.

Seasonal Vegetable Platter: A vibrant assortment of locally-sourced, organic vegetables served with a homemade hummus dip.

Main Course:

Roasted Pumpkin Risotto: A creamy risotto made with pumpkin, sage, and Parmesan, symbolizing warmth and comfort.

Grilled Portobello Mushrooms: Marinated in balsamic and garlic, representing the earthy connection of the group.

Side Dishes:

Quinoa and Roasted Beet Salad: Colorful beets and fluffy quinoa dressed in a citrus vinaigrette, showcasing nature's bounty.

Sautéed Green Beans with Almonds: Fresh green beans lightly sautéed and topped with crunchy almonds.

Dessert:

Fig and Honey Tart: Sweet figs drizzled with honey on a delicate pastry crust, embodying the sweetness of life.

Artisanal Cheese Board: A selection of fine cheeses, accompanied by nuts and fruit, encouraging shared tastes and experiences.

Beverages:

Local Wine Selection: Carefully chosen wines from the surrounding vineyards of the Mornington Peninsula.

Herbal Infusion Tea: A soothing blend of herbs from the garden, perfect for winding down the evening.

Eternal Flames

Vegan Tantric Feast Menu

Appetisers:
Grilled Vegetable Bruschetta: Char-grilled seasonal vegetables on toasted sourdough, drizzled with balsamic glaze.
Stuffed Dates with Almond Butter: Medjool dates filled with creamy almond butter, a sweet and savory delight.

Main Course:
Coconut Curry with Seasonal Vegetables: Aromatic and creamy coconut curry loaded with fresh, local vegetables.
Stuffed Bell Peppers: Bell peppers filled with quinoa, black beans, and spices, baked to perfection.

Side Dishes:
Kale and Avocado Salad: Massaged kale salad with avocado slices, pumpkin seeds, and a lemon-tahini dressing.
Roasted Sweet Potato Wedges: Seasoned with herbs and served with a homemade vegan aioli.

Dessert:
Raw Chocolate and Nut Tart: A decadent, no-bake tart made with raw cacao and assorted nuts.
Fruit Platter: An assortment of fresh, seasonal fruits to cleanse the palate.

Beverages:
Homemade Lemon and Mint Iced Tea: Refreshing and invigorating, perfect for cleansing the palate.
Organic Red and White Wines: A selection of vegan-friendly wines from local vineyards.

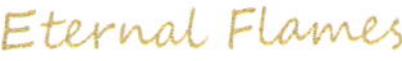

9: Across Seas and Souls

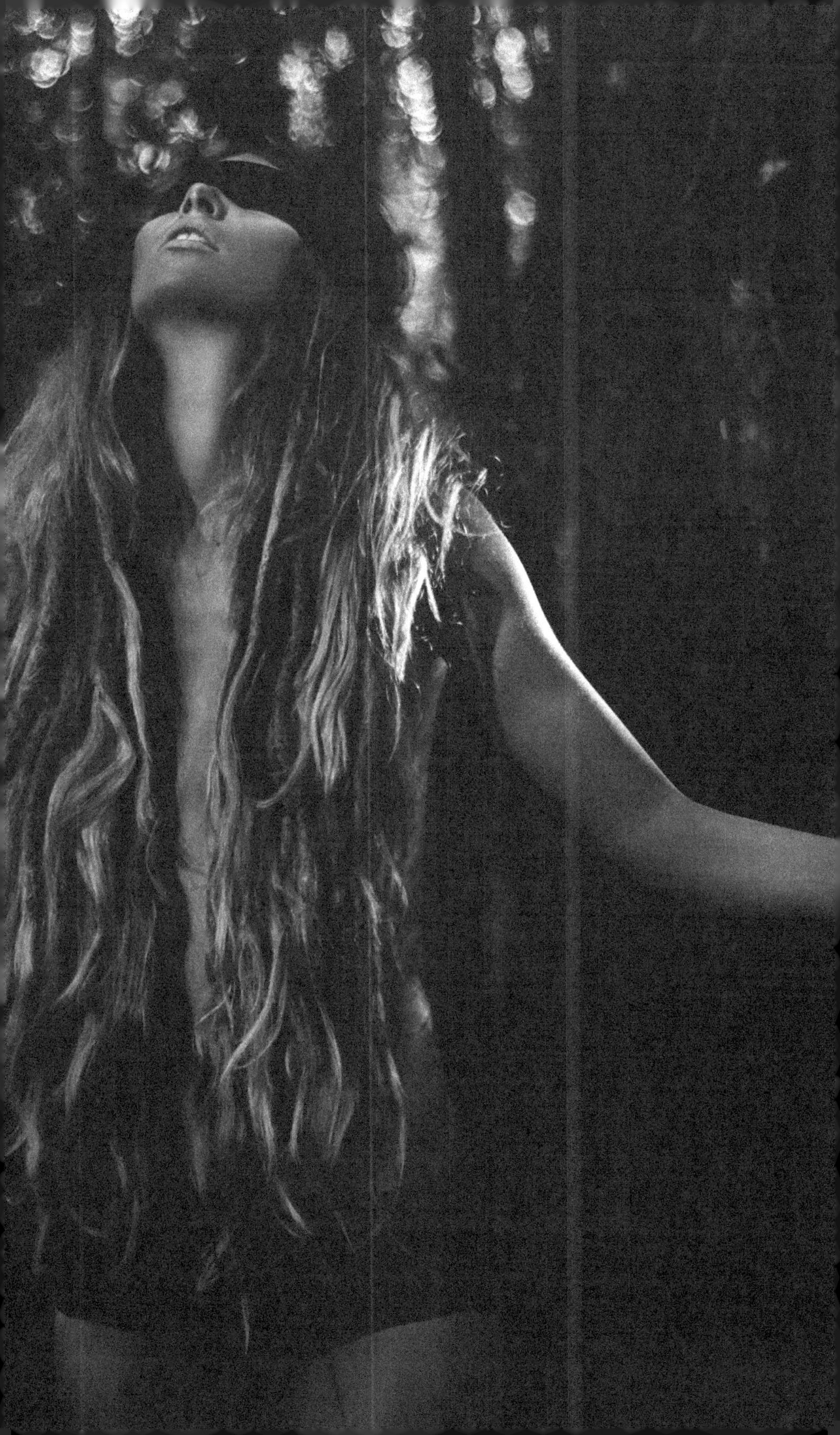

Chapter 9: Across Seas and Souls

Ethan gazed out of his hotel room window at the bustling streets of Paris, his thoughts drifting thousands of miles to the cozy cottage on the Mornington Peninsula, where Mia, his soulmate, waited. It had been three weeks since he left for his work trip across Europe, and each day the distance seemed to grow heavier, a tangible weight on his heart.

Tonight, they had planned to bridge this gap with a long-distance tantric ritual, a practice they hoped would renew their connection, despite the miles separating them. Ethan prepared his room, dimming the lights and lighting a small candle, its flame flickering like a distant star in the evening sky.

Back home, Mia was doing the same, her heart fluttering with anticipation. The soft glow of candlelight filled their living room, casting a warm, golden light that seemed to hold Ethan's essence. She positioned her laptop on the coffee table, the portal through which Ethan would join her.

As the clock struck their agreed-upon time, Ethan's face appeared on Mia's screen, a comforting sight that brought an immediate smile to her face. Their eyes met through the digital ether, a connection that transcended the physical, a testament to their deep, unspoken bond.

They began with the opening connection, sharing their intentions for the practice. "I want to feel close to you, to bridge this distance even if just for a moment," Ethan said, his voice laced with emotion. Mia echoed his sentiment, expressing her longing to feel his presence, to remember the strength of their bond. Moving into synchronised breathing, they closed their eyes, inhaling and exhaling in unison.
The sound of their breaths, harmonised through the speakers, created an intimate rhythm, a dance of air and spirit that wove them together across the continents.

Ethan then led a guided visualisation, describing a cherished memory of a day they had spent together on a secluded beach in Australia.
Mia's imagination took flight, and soon she could almost feel the

sun's warmth on her skin, the sand beneath her feet, Ethan's hand in hers.

In the energy connection exercise, they focused on their heart chakras, visualizing a radiant energy that spanned the distance between them. Mia pictured a vibrant thread of light, a connection that pulsed with love and longing, reaching out to Ethan.

They recited their chosen mantra, "Together in heart, always," a powerful affirmation that echoed in their shared virtual space. With each repetition, their voices blended, reinforcing their bond, a reminder that their love knew no bounds.

As they concluded the practice, they shared their experiences and feelings. Ethan spoke of a profound sense of closeness, as if Mia were right there with him. Mia shared the warmth and comfort she had felt, the visualization bringing Ethan's presence to life.

They ended the session with heartfelt messages, promises of love and reunion. As they said their goodbyes, Ethan blew out his candle, the smoke rising and disappearing, a symbol of their ephemeral yet eternal connection.

Ethan lay in bed that night, the distance feeling a little less daunting. In his heart, he carried the warmth of their ritual, a reminder that no matter how far he travelled, Mia was always with him, a constant presence in his soul.

Back in the cottage, Mia watched the candle's flame dwindle, feeling a sense of peace. The ritual had been a balm to her longing, a bridge across the ocean, bringing Ethan's spirit home to her, if only for a while.

As they both drifted to sleep in their respective worlds, they were united by a profound understanding – their love was a journey, not of miles, but of souls, a journey that continued to unfold, no matter the distance.

Long Distance Ritual

A tantric practice for a long-distance relationship involves adapting traditional elements of tantra to a virtual environment. The focus remains on emotional and spiritual connection, using tools like synchronised activities, visualisation and shared intentions to bridge the physical gap.

Total Duration: 30 - 45 minutes

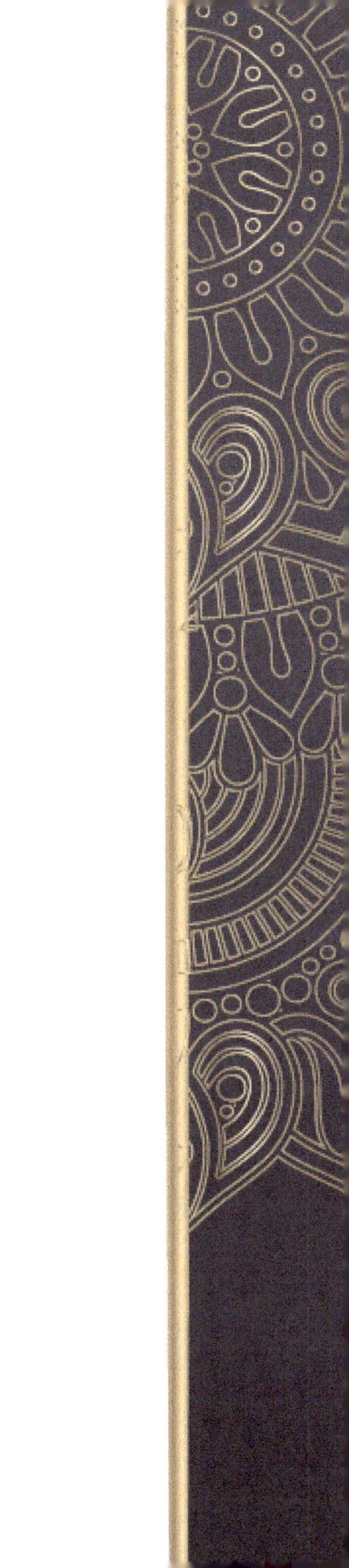

Preparation:
Schedule a time when both partners are free from
distractions and can fully engage in the practice.
Each partner creates a comfortable and serene space in
their respective locations. This can include dimming the
lights, lighting candles, and perhaps playing soft, ambient
music.

Opening Connection (5 minutes):
Begin with a video call. Start by looking into each other's
eyes through the screen, trying to maintain a soft and
loving gaze, just as you would in person.

Share your intentions for the practice, speaking about what
you hope to achieve or feel. This might include deepening
your emotional connection, fostering intimacy, or simply
being present with each other.

Synchronised Breathing (5-10 minutes):
Close your eyes and guide each other through deep,
synchronised breathing. Inhale and exhale together, trying
to match the length and depth of each other's breaths.
Use the sound of your partner's breath over the call as a
guide, allowing this shared rhythm to create a sense of
closeness.

Guided Visualisation (10 minutes):
One partner leads a guided visualisation. Imagine a
place where you both feel happy and at peace, perhaps
somewhere you've been together or a place you dream of
visiting.
Describe the sensations you feel in this shared space – the
sights, sounds, and smells. Allow yourselves to feel as though
you are both truly there together.

Energy Connection Exercise (5-10 minutes):
Focus on the heart chakra, located in the center of the
chest. Feel a glowing light or energy radiating from this
space.

Imagine this energy reaching out across the distance, connecting with your partner's heart chakra. See your energies mingling and swirling together in a harmonious dance.

Shared Mantra or Affirmation (5 minutes):
Choose a mantra or affirmation to recite together. This could be something like, "Our love knows no distance" or "Together in heart, always".
Repeat the mantra several times together, allowing its meaning to resonate deeply within both of you.

Closing the Practice (5 minutes):
Share any feelings, sensations, or thoughts that came up during the practice.
Express gratitude for each other and for the technology that allows you to connect in this way.

Conclude with a loving or inspirational message to each other, carrying the sense of connection forward.

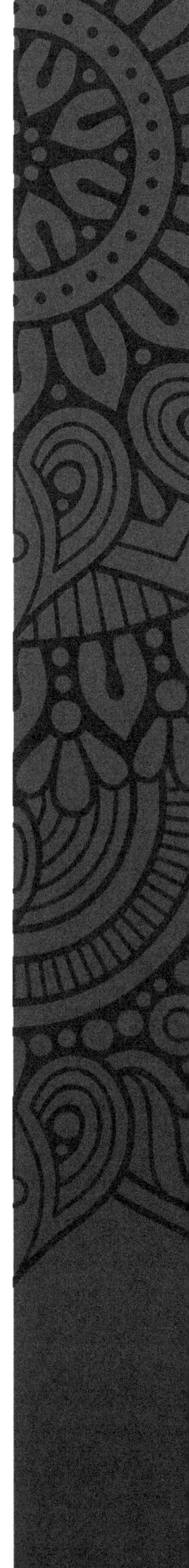

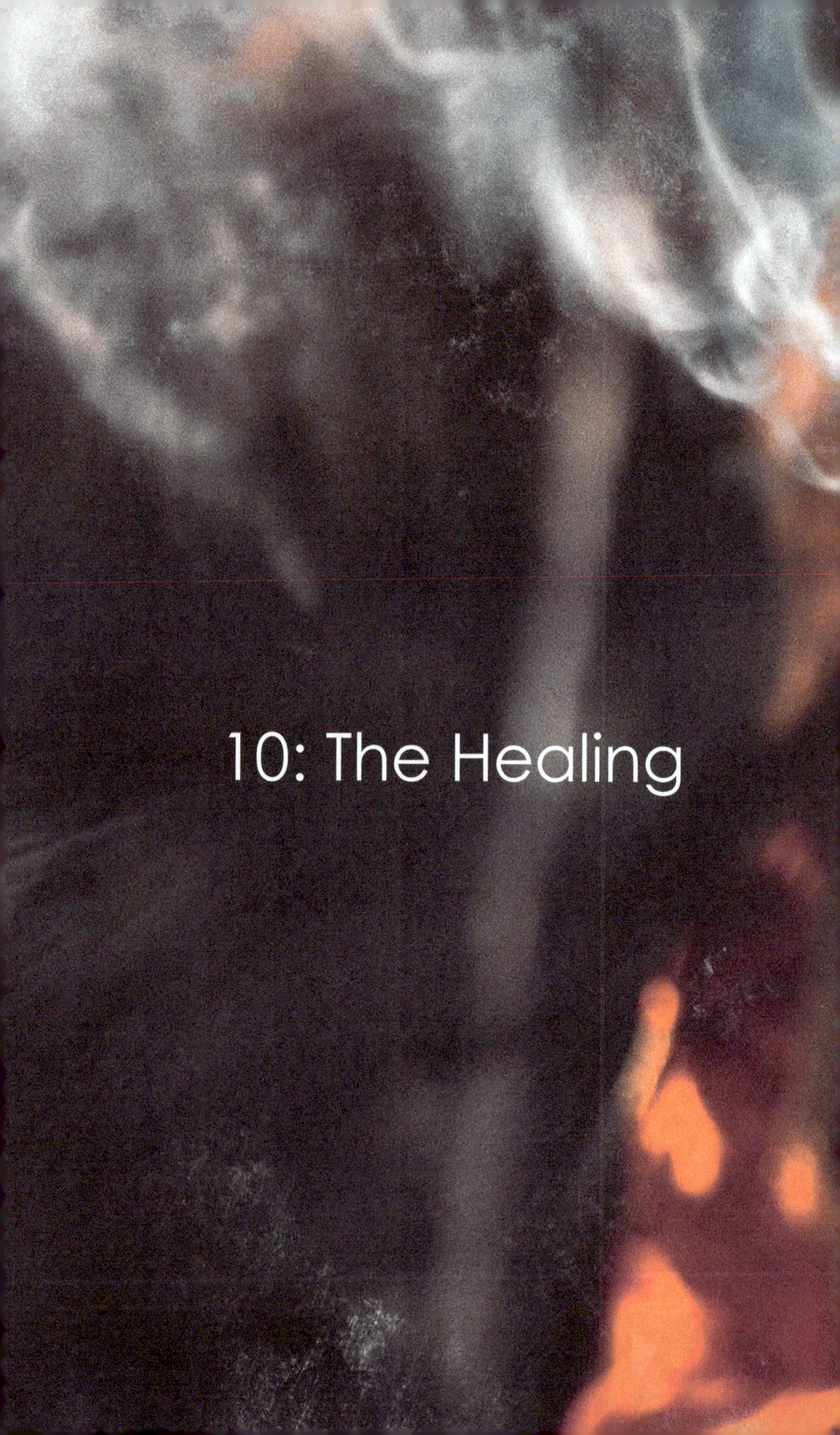
10: The Healing

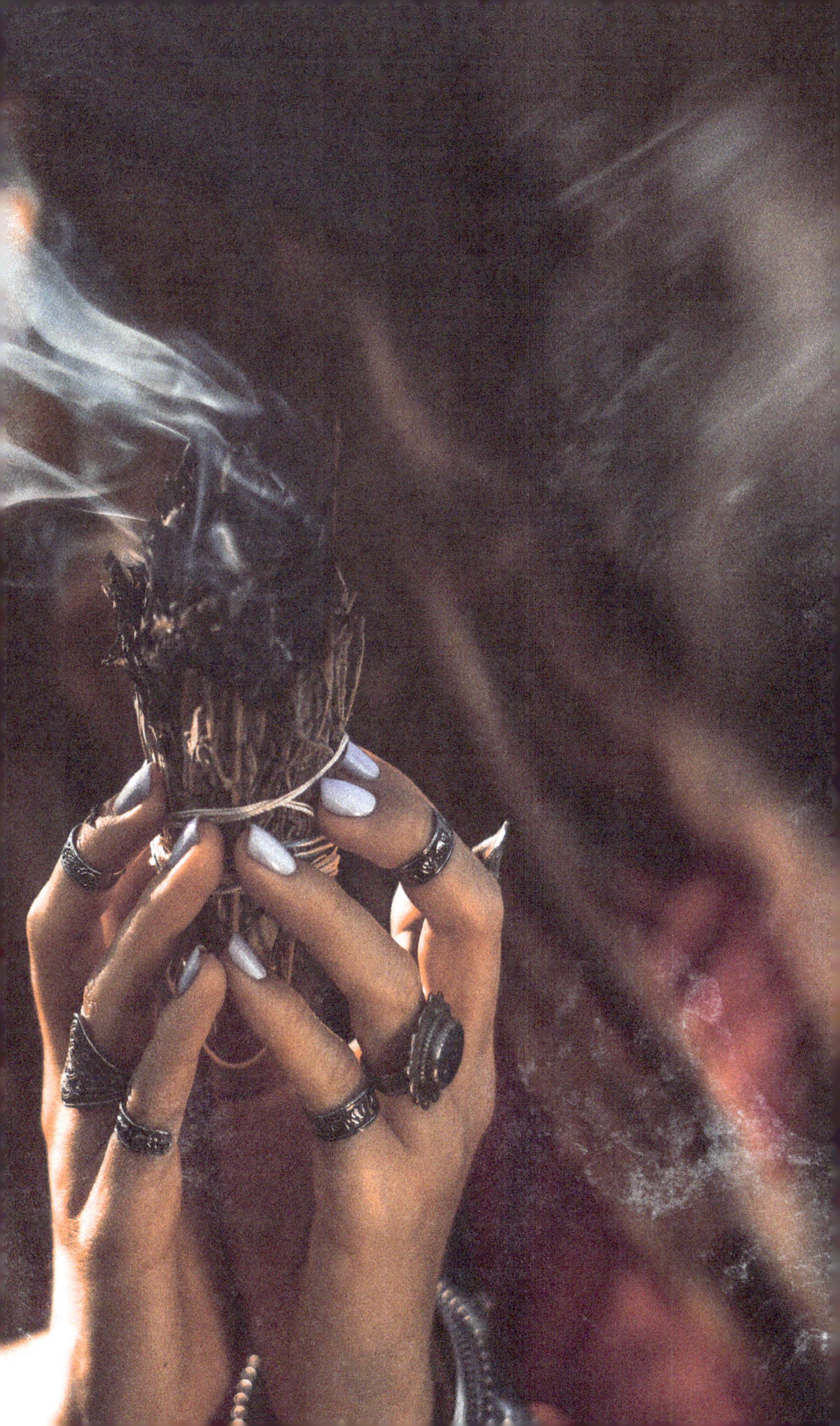

Chapter 10: The Healing Dance

Mia's illness had cast a shadow over the once vibrant cottage, her recovery slow and arduous. The days that used to be filled with laughter and shared adventures were now quieter, more reflective.
Ethan, ever the pillar of strength and love, stood steadfastly by her side, yet he too felt the weight of worry and helplessness.

Seeking to bring back the light into their lives and speed Mia's healing, Ethan reached out to Aria, their trusted tantric healer, a woman of profound wisdom and kindness.
Aria had been a guiding force in their spiritual journey and Ethan hoped her expertise in tantric healing could aid Mia's recovery.

Aria arrived at the cottage on a cool autumn afternoon, her presence immediately filling the space with a sense of calm and hope. After a heartfelt reunion, they prepared the living room for the healing ritual.
Aria instructed them to create a circle with cushions, placing candles and crystals at specific points to align with earth's energy fields.

As they settled into the circle, Aria began with a gentle meditation, guiding Mia and Ethan to visualise healing energy surrounding them.
Mia, her energy still frail, closed her eyes and focused on the soothing cadence of Aria's voice, feeling a sense of peace enveloping her.

Aria then moved to the chakra balancing part of the ritual. She used a combination of sound therapy with Tibetan singing bowls and guided visualisation to help align and open Mia's chakras, focusing particularly on the heart and solar plexus chakras, which are centers of healing and energy.

With each chime of the bowls, Mia felt a gentle wave of vibrations flowing through her, easing the tension and fatigue that had become her constant companions.
Ethan, sitting beside her, held her hand, his own energy focused on sending love and strength to her.

Next came the practice of synchronised breathing. Aria instructed Ethan to match his breathing with Mia's more shallow breaths. This exercise, Aria explained, was not just about physical synchronisation, but about Ethan lending his strength and vitality to Mia. As they breathed together, Mia felt a surge of energy, as if Ethan's breath was indeed filling her with life and vigour.

Aria then moved on to a gentle tantric massage, using essential oils to massage Mia's feet, hands, and head. The touch was healing, filled with intention and care. Mia's body, which had been tensed with discomfort, began to relax, the pain ebbing away under Aria's skilled hands.

As the ritual neared its end, Aria led them in a mantra chanting, choosing words that evoked healing and strength. Their voices, joined in unison, filled the room, creating a harmonious symphony of sound and intention. Mia's voice, weak at first, grew stronger with each repetition, a testament to the energy flowing back into her.

Finally, Aria concluded the ritual with a closing meditation, enveloping the room in a sense of gratitude and peace. As they opened their eyes, Mia and Ethan shared a look of profound love and thankfulness. Mia, though still on her path to recovery, felt a renewed sense of hope and strength.

Aria left them with words of wisdom, reminding them that healing is as much a journey of the spirit as it is of the body. As night fell, the cottage, now imbued with the residual energy of the ritual, seemed to glow with a newfound light.

Ethan and Mia, nestled together, felt a deep sense of gratitude. The ritual had been a balm to their weary spirits, a reminder of the healing power of love, connection, and the ancient wisdom of tantra.
They knew the road ahead might still hold challenges, but they also knew they had the strength and love to face them, together.

A Healing Ritual

This ritual is designed to aid in recovery from a prolonged illness, focusing on restoring balance, energy, and well-being. It combines elements of meditation, energy work, and affirmations, tailored for healing and rejuvenation.

Total Duration: 45-60 minutes

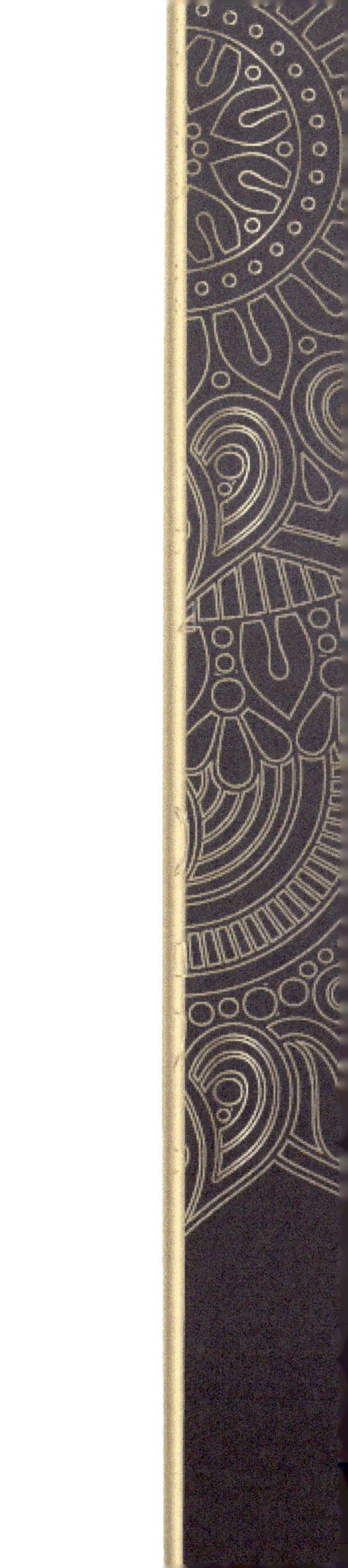

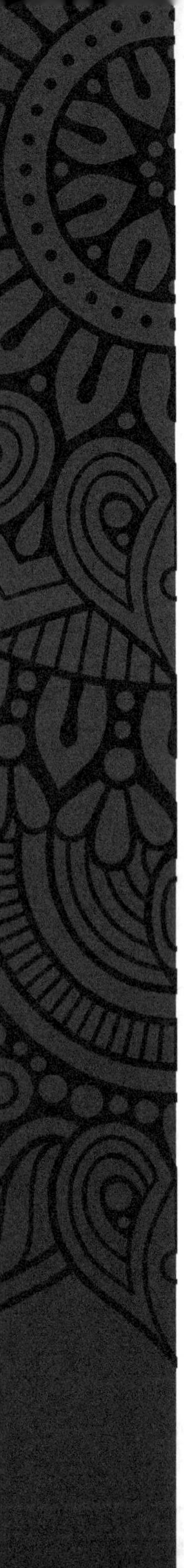

Preparation:
Find a quiet and comfortable space where you won't be disturbed. You may sit or lie down on a cushion or yoga mat.
Light candles or incense to create a peaceful atmosphere. Optionally, play soft, soothing music in the background.

Grounding and Centering (5 minutes):
Deep Breathing: Begin with deep, slow breaths to center yourself. Inhale deeply through your nose, filling your lungs completely, and exhale slowly through your mouth. This helps in releasing tension and grounding your energy

Body Scan Meditation: Gently shift your focus to different parts of your body, starting from your toes and moving upwards. As you focus on each part, breathe into it, allowing relaxation and release of any discomfort.

Chakra Balancing (10 minutes):
Focus on Each Chakra: Starting from the root chakra at the base of the spine, focus on each of the seven chakras. Visualise a healing light or energy at each chakra, imagining it balancing and rejuvenating the chakra.

Chanting Mantras: For each chakra, softly chant or mentally recite a corresponding Bija mantra (LAM for Root, VAM for Sacral, RAM for Solar Plexus, YAM for Heart, HAM for Throat, OM for Third Eye, and AH for Crown). This helps in aligning and harmonising the energy centers.

Healing Visualisation (10 minutes):
Visualise Healing Energy: Imagine a healing light or energy engulfing your body, starting from your feet and moving upwards. Visualize this light healing and restoring every cell in your body.

Affirmations: Repeat healing affirmations such as "I am healing", "My body is strong and healthy", or "With every breath, I am restoring my well-being."

Reconnecting with Nature (5 minutes):
Earth Connection: If possible, briefly step outside barefoot to connect with the earth or simply visualize this connection. Feel the energy of the earth supporting and nourishing your body.

Closing the Ritual (5 minutes):
Gratitude: Finish the ritual with a moment of gratitude. Acknowledge your body's strength and resilience, and express thanks for the healing journey.

Gentle Transition: Slowly bring your awareness back to the present moment. Gently move your fingers and toes, stretch if needed, and open your eyes when ready.

This ritual should be approached with gentle intention and self-compassion, allowing the body and mind to embrace the healing process at their own pace. It can be repeated as often as needed to aid in recovery and rejuvenation.

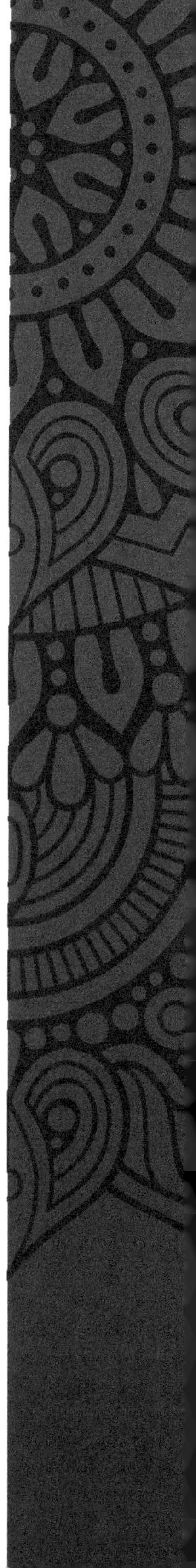

12: Embracing the Elements

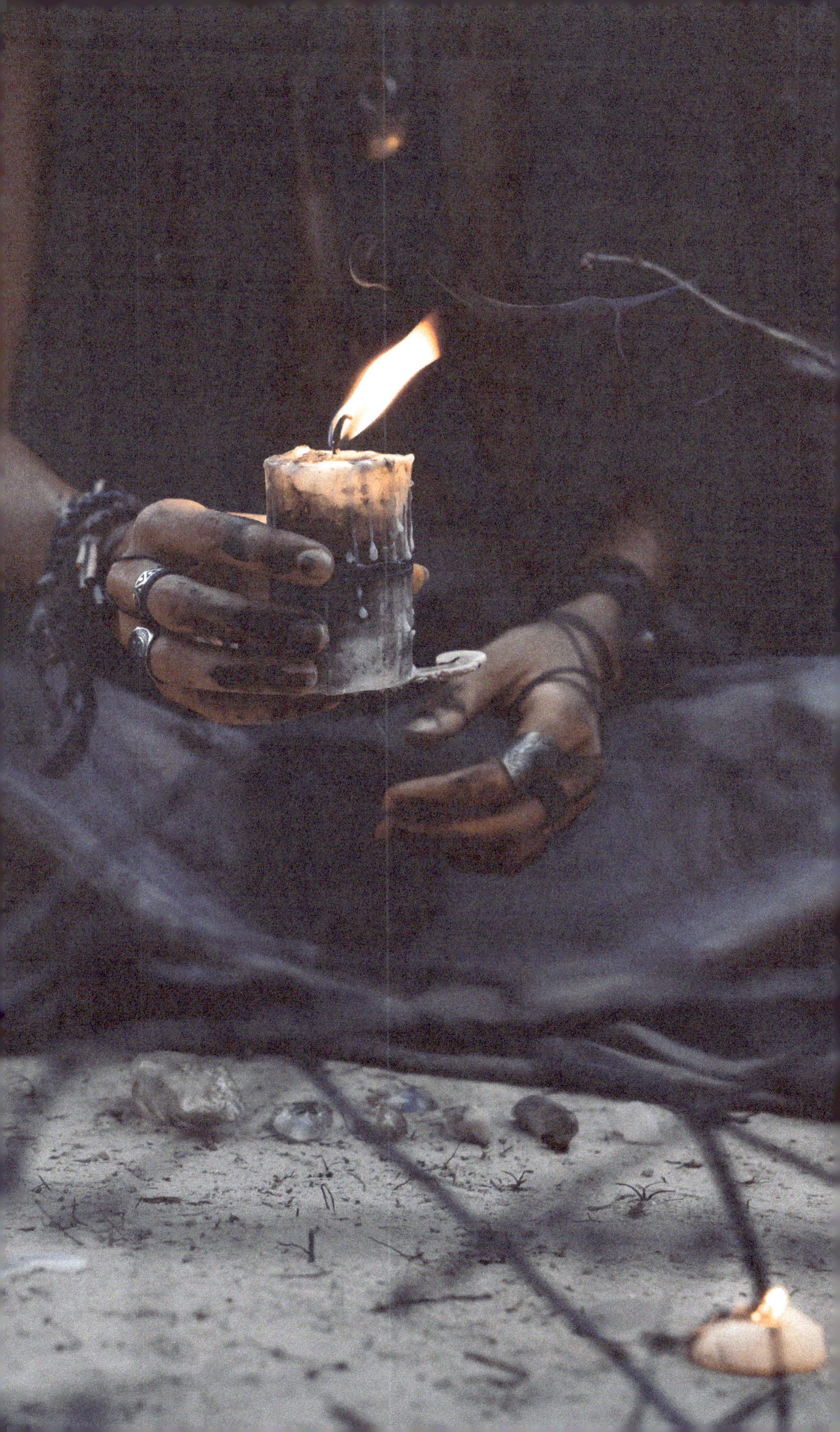

Chapter 12: Embracing the Elements

Mia stood in the heart of her beloved cottage, transformed tonight into a sanctuary for the Women's Circle she had gathered. Her journey of healing had rekindled in her a desire to connect more deeply with the women in her life – friends who had become her sisters in spirit. This evening, they were to partake in a Four Elements Ritual, a practice Mia had carefully chosen for its grounding and empowering energy.

The living room was a haven of tranquility and strength. In the center, a large, circular mat lay surrounded by cushions, each placed thoughtfully for her friends. In the cardinal directions of the circle, Mia had set symbols representing the four elements: a potted plant for Earth in the north, a bowl of water for Water in the west, candles for Fire in the south, and several incense sticks for Air in the east.

As the women arrived, each was greeted with a warm embrace. They settled into the circle, a sense of anticipation and camaraderie filling the air. Mia, her heart full, began the ritual with a moment of silent gratitude for the gathering of these remarkable women.

She guided them first to the Earth element. They held the soil from the potted plant, feeling its texture and solidity. Mia spoke of the Earth's nurturing and sustaining qualities, inviting each woman to share a moment when they felt supported or grounded. The stories woven were rich tapestries of resilience and strength.

Next was the Water element. They passed the bowl, each woman touching the water, reflecting on its fluidity and adaptability. Mia encouraged them to contemplate times when they had adapted to change or had to be fluid in their thoughts or actions. Their shared experiences created ripples of empathy and understanding in the circle.

Moving to the Fire element, Mia lit the candles, the flames casting a warm, reassuring glow. Fire, she explained, was about passion, energy, and transformation. The women discussed moments of personal transformation, their passions and dreams, the light of the flames mirroring the fire in their stories and in their hearts.

Lastly, they focused on the Air element, the incense filling the room with a gentle, fragrant smoke. Air, Mia noted, was about thoughts, communication, and the spirit. The women took turns speaking about their hopes, their wisdom, and the power of their voices, each story a breath of inspiration.

As the ritual drew to a close, Mia led the circle in a meditation, visualizing the harmonious blending of the four elements within themselves. They imagined drawing strength from the Earth, embracing the fluidity of Water, igniting the fire of their passions, and letting their thoughts and spirit soar like the Air.

The Women's Circle concluded with each woman expressing gratitude for the shared experience and for the support they found in one another. Hugs and smiles were exchanged, the air thick with a sense of unity and empowerment.

After her friends had departed, Mia sat alone for a moment, the remnants of the ritual around her. She felt a profound connection to the elements, to her friends, and to herself.
Tonight, the Women's Circle had not just been a gathering; it had been a celebration of the elemental forces within and around them, a testament to the strength and beauty of the feminine spirit.

In the quiet of the cottage, Mia felt a deep sense of peace.
The Four Elements Ritual had been a journey of connection, a reminder of the power that lay in unity and in the sacred dance of the elements.
As she blew out the candles, she knew this was just the beginning of many more gatherings, each a chance to explore, share, and grow in the company of extraordinary women.

Women's Circle Full Moon Ritual with Opening of the Four Elements

This ritual is designed for a Women's Circle to celebrate and harness the energy of the full moon, beginning with an acknowledgment of the four elements – Earth, Water, Fire, and Air. It's a time for reflection, release, and setting intentions.

Total Duration: 60- 90 minutes

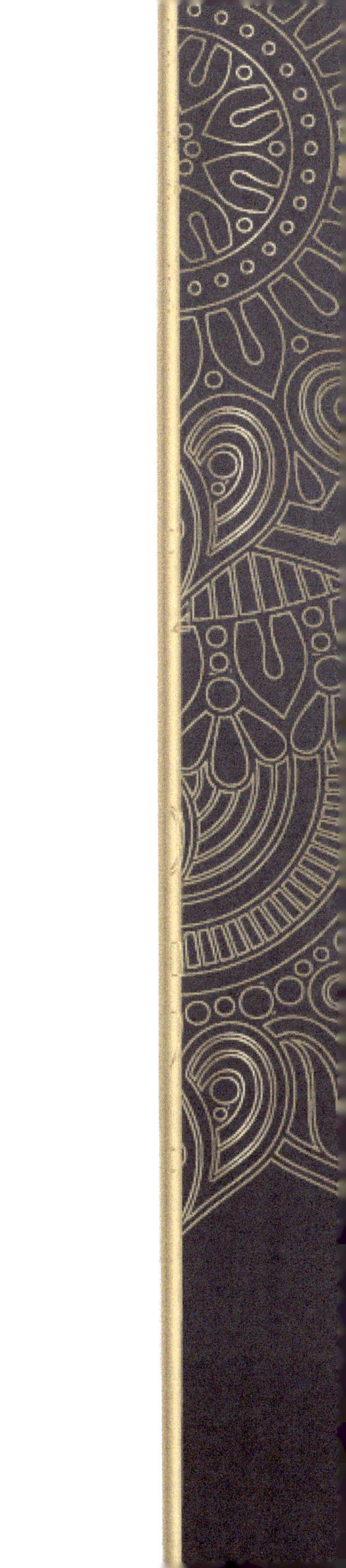

Preparation:
Create a Sacred Space: Choose a quiet and comfortable outdoor or indoor space where the group can sit in a circle. If indoors, ensure the room is airy and has enough space.
Altar Set-Up: In the center of the circle, set up a small altar with symbols representing the four elements: a bowl of soil or a plant for Earth, a bowl of water for Water, candles for Fire, and incense for Air.

Opening Ceremony (10 minutes):
Welcoming the Four Elements: Begin by acknowledging the four elements. Pass around the bowl of soil, the bowl of water, and then light the candles and incense, allowing each participant to feel or interact with these elements as they are passed around.

Setting Intentions: Invite each participant to share their intention for the ritual or something they wish to release or manifest with the full moon's energy.

Grounding and Centering (5 minutes):
Guided Grounding Meditation: Lead a short meditation to ground and center the group. Encourage everyone to visualize roots growing from the base of their spine into the earth, connecting deeply with Earth's energy.

Full Moon Reflections (15 minutes):
Sharing Circle: Under the light of the full moon, invite each woman to share her reflections on the past lunar cycle – challenges, achievements, or insights. This is a time for listening and holding space for each other.

Releasing Ceremony (10 minutes):
Writing and Release: Hand out pieces of paper and pens. Ask each woman to write down what they wish to release with this full moon. One by one, have them throw their papers into a fire-safe bowl and burn them, symbolizing the release of these energies.

Setting New Intentions (10 minutes):

Manifestation Exercise: Guide the group to silently set new intentions for the coming lunar cycle. They can focus on what they wish to attract or manifest.

Full Moon Energy Work (10 minutes):

Full Moon Visualisation: Lead a visualisation where everyone imagines bathing in the silver light of the full moon, absorbing its energy, and filling themselves with clarity, peace, and strength.

Closing Ceremony (10 minutes):

Thanking the Four Elements: Close the ritual by thanking the four elements for their presence and support. Extinguish the candles and incense, symbolizing the end of the ritual.

Group Hug or Handhold: Conclude with a group hug or by holding hands, affirming the unity and shared energy of the circle.

Post-Ritual:

Sharing Food and Drink: After the ritual, share some light refreshments. This is a time for informal conversation and grounding before leaving the space.

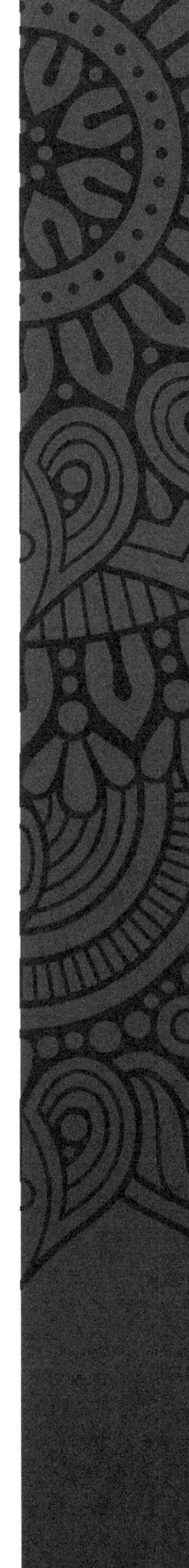

10 Centrepiece Ideas utilising the Four Elements

Nature's Mandala: Arrange leaves, flowers, stones, and shells in a mandala pattern, symbolizing the unity of the elements.

Candle and Crystals Grid: Place candles for Fire, surrounded by crystals representing Earth, bowls of water, and feather for Air.

Seasonal Altar: Decorate with seasonal natural elements like autumn leaves, spring flowers, summer fruits, and winter branches.

Elemental Jars: Create four jars filled with items representing each element – soil for Earth, water with floating flowers for Water, candles for Fire, and incense for Air.

Beach Theme: Use sand, shells, and seawater for a beach-themed altar, with a small fire pit or candles and a gentle breeze or fan for Air.

Herbal Circle: A ring of different herbs for Earth, with a central bowl of water, candles, and incense sticks.

Rustic Wooden Tray: A wooden tray with a moss bed (Earth), small water vessel, candle holder, and an airy, light feather or incense.

Four Corners Altar: Set up the altar in four sections, each dedicated to one element, using items like rocks, shells, candles, and feathers.

Garden Inspired: Utilise potted plants, fresh water in a clear vase, a small campfire or candle arrangement, and wind chimes.

Floating Elements: A large bowl of water with floating candles (Fire), stones (Earth), and flower petals (Air).

Creating Your Altar

Creating a centrepiece or altar for a women's circle is a wonderful way to set a sacred and welcoming space.

The altar is a living, breathing part of Circles, evolving with each gathering. It's not just about aesthetics - it's a reflection of the collective energy, intentions and spirits of the participants.
Approach your next altar or centrepiece with creativity, respect and mindfulness throughout the process.

Choosing Items
Your altar should be a reflection of the Earth and the group's collective spirit. Incorporate natural elements such as flowers, stones, crystals, or water to symbolise your connection to nature.
Personal objects like photographs, keepsakes, or artworks add a layer of individual significance. Candles and incense can be used to create a serene atmosphere, but always be mindful of safety and allergies. If appropriate, include cultural or spiritual symbols, ensuring they are used with respect and understanding of their origins and meanings.

Arrangement
The arrangement of your altar is key to creating a harmonious and accessible space. Arrange items so they are visible to all members, perhaps in a circular or symmetrical pattern that represents unity and balance. Strive for a visual balance in colours, textures, and sizes of objects to create a harmonious and inviting space.

Participation
Encourage each participant to contribute an item to the altar. This act fosters a sense of community and shared ownership. Invite participants to share the significance of their items, deepening the group's connection and understanding.

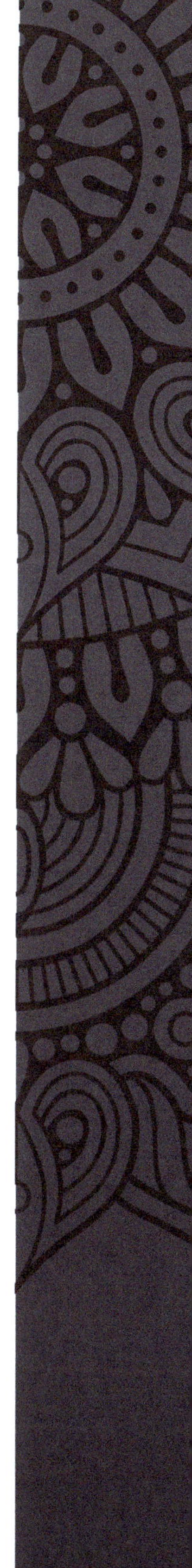

13: The Circle of Elements and Brotherhood

Chapter 13: The Circle of Elements and Brotherhood

As the first blossoms of spring adorned the vineyards, Ethan prepared for a gathering that held a special place in his heart.

He had invited his closest male friends to join him for a Men's Circle, a space for sharing, reflection, and connection. Tonight, they would engage in a Four Elements Ritual, drawing on the powerful symbolism of Earth, Water, Fire, and Air to deepen their bond and understanding.

In the open expanse of Ethan's property, under the vast, starlit sky, a fire pit crackled with welcoming flames, embodying the Fire element. Around it, Ethan had set up four stations, each representing one of the elements.
For Earth, there was a collection of stones and soil; for Water, a bowl of clear spring water; and for Air, an open space marked by fluttering flags. The Fire element was the heart of their gathering, the fire pit around which they would all sit.

As his friends arrived, each carrying their own stories and experiences, the atmosphere was one of camaraderie and anticipation. Among them were Alex with his drum and Liam with his guitar, their instruments adding a layer of primal energy to the night.

The circle began with each man taking a moment to stand at the Earth station, holding a stone or handful of soil. Ethan spoke of stability, growth, and resilience. They reflected on times they had felt grounded or needed to be strong like the Earth. The soft thrum of Alex's drum underscored their shared reflections.

Next, they moved to the Water station. Here, each man touched the water, contemplating its fluidity and the ability to adapt. They shared experiences of change and emotional depth, the water symbolising the flow of life and the importance of emotional fluidity in their journey as men.

The Fire was the central element of their ritual. Gathered around the blazing pit, they spoke of passion, transformation, and energy

Liam strummed his guitar, creating a warm melody that danced with the flames. The men shared stories of personal challenges, ambitions, and the fires that drove them. In the glow of the fire, their faces were etched with the sincerity of their words.
Lastly, they stood in the space marked for Air, feeling the gentle spring breeze.
This was a time to reflect on thoughts, communication, and spirituality. They discussed their hopes, ideas, and the power of their voices in their communities and families.
The music of the guitar and drum floated up into the night, mingling with their spoken truths.

As the ritual drew to a close, Ethan led them in a meditation, visualizing the harmonious integration of the elements within themselves. They imagined drawing strength from the Earth, embracing the adaptability of Water, fuelling the inner fire of their passions, and letting their spirits soar with the Air.

The Men's Circle concluded with a powerful drum and guitar session, the rhythm and melodies echoing the heartbeat of their shared experience. As they packed up, there was a palpable sense of unity and brotherhood.

Ethan watched his friends leave, feeling a profound gratitude for the night. The Four Elements Ritual had not just been a gathering; it had been a journey of connection to the natural world and to each other. In the embers of the dying fire, he saw the reflection of their bond – strong, warm, and enduring.

As he walked back to the cottage, Ethan carried with him the energy and lessons of the night. The Men's Circle under the spring sky had been a celebration of masculinity in its most genuine form, a space where strength was measured not just in physical might, but in vulnerability, honesty, and the courage to connect.

Men's Circle Fire Ritual with the Four Elements

This ritual is tailored for an adult men's circle, designed to be held around a fire, incorporating the four elements (Earth, Water, Fire, Air) and the use of drums. It's a space for connection, introspection, and sharing, aimed at fostering brotherhood and personal growth.

Total Duration: 60 - 90 minutes

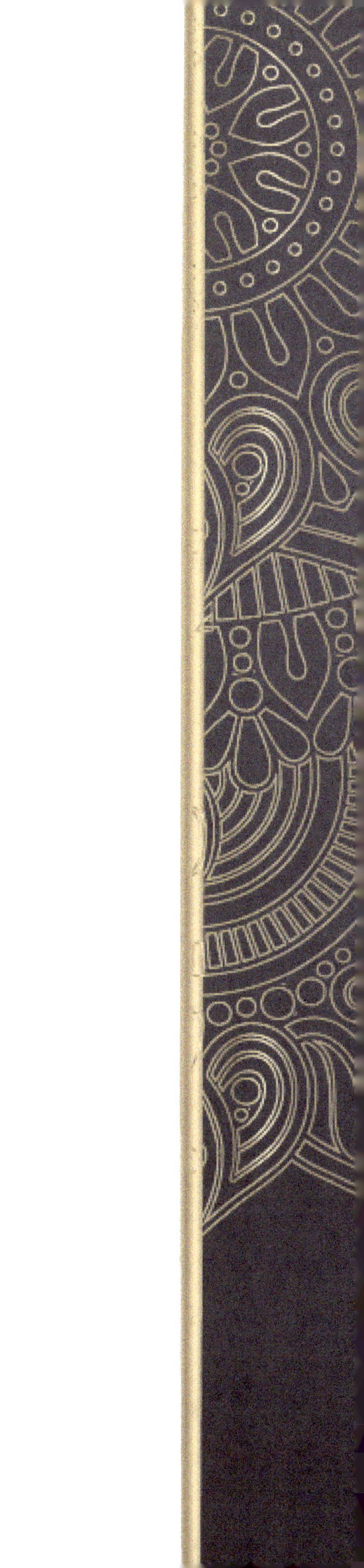

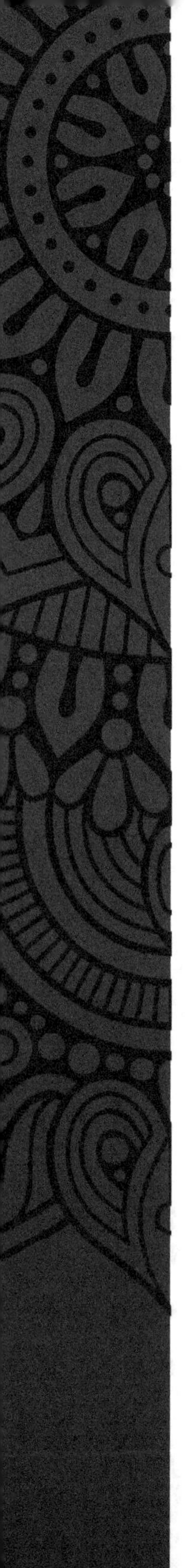

Preparation:

Create a Sacred Space: Choose an outdoor space where a safe fire can be lit. Arrange seating in a circle around the fire pit.

Altar Set-Up: Near the fire, set up a small altar with symbols of the four elements: a bowl of soil or stones for Earth, a bowl of water for Water, the fire pit for Fire, and feathers or incense for Air.

Drums and Instruments: Place drums and any other percussion instruments near the circle for participants to use during the ritual.

Opening Ceremony (15 minutes):

Welcoming the Four Elements: Begin by acknowledging each of the four elements. Pass around the bowl of soil or stones, the bowl of water, light the fire, and then light the incense, allowing each man to interact with these elements.

Setting Intentions: Invite each participant to share an intention for the evening or something they are seeking from the ritual – be it guidance, strength, or release.

Drumming and Grounding (10 minutes):

Rhythmic Drumming: Start a rhythmic drumming session, encouraging each participant to join in. The drumming helps in grounding and connecting with the Earth's energy.

Guided Grounding Exercise: Lead a short meditation, focusing on the rhythm of the drumbeats, imagining roots growing from each person's feet deep into the earth.

Fire Gazing Meditation (15 minutes):

Silent Reflection: Guide the group to gaze into the fire silently, contemplating the transformative power of Fire. This serves as a meditation for introspection and inner clarity.

Sharing Circle: After the meditation, those who feel moved

to share insights or reflections prompted by the fire gazing can do so.

Water Cleansing Ritual (10 minutes):
Purification and Release: Use the bowl of water in a cleansing ritual. Each man can wash his hands in the water, symbolizing the washing away of old energies, patterns, or burdens.

Air Element – Breathing Exercise (10 minutes):
Breathwork for Release: Lead a breathing exercise focusing on the Air element. Instruct the group to take deep breaths, visualizing clarity and lightness with each inhale and exhale.
Affirmations: Introduce a round of affirmations or positive statements that each man can say aloud, harnessing the power of spoken words.

Closing Ceremony (10 minutes):
Thanking the Elements: Conclude by thanking each of the four elements for their guidance and energy.
Closing the Circle: End the ritual by acknowledging the brotherhood and the shared experience, possibly with a group chant or a moment of silence.

Post-Ritual:
Sharing Food and Drink: Offer light refreshments after the ritual. This time can be used for casual conversation, allowing the group to transition back from the ritual space.

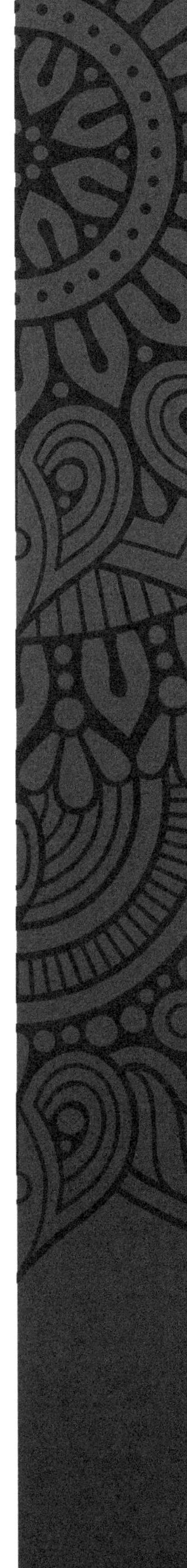

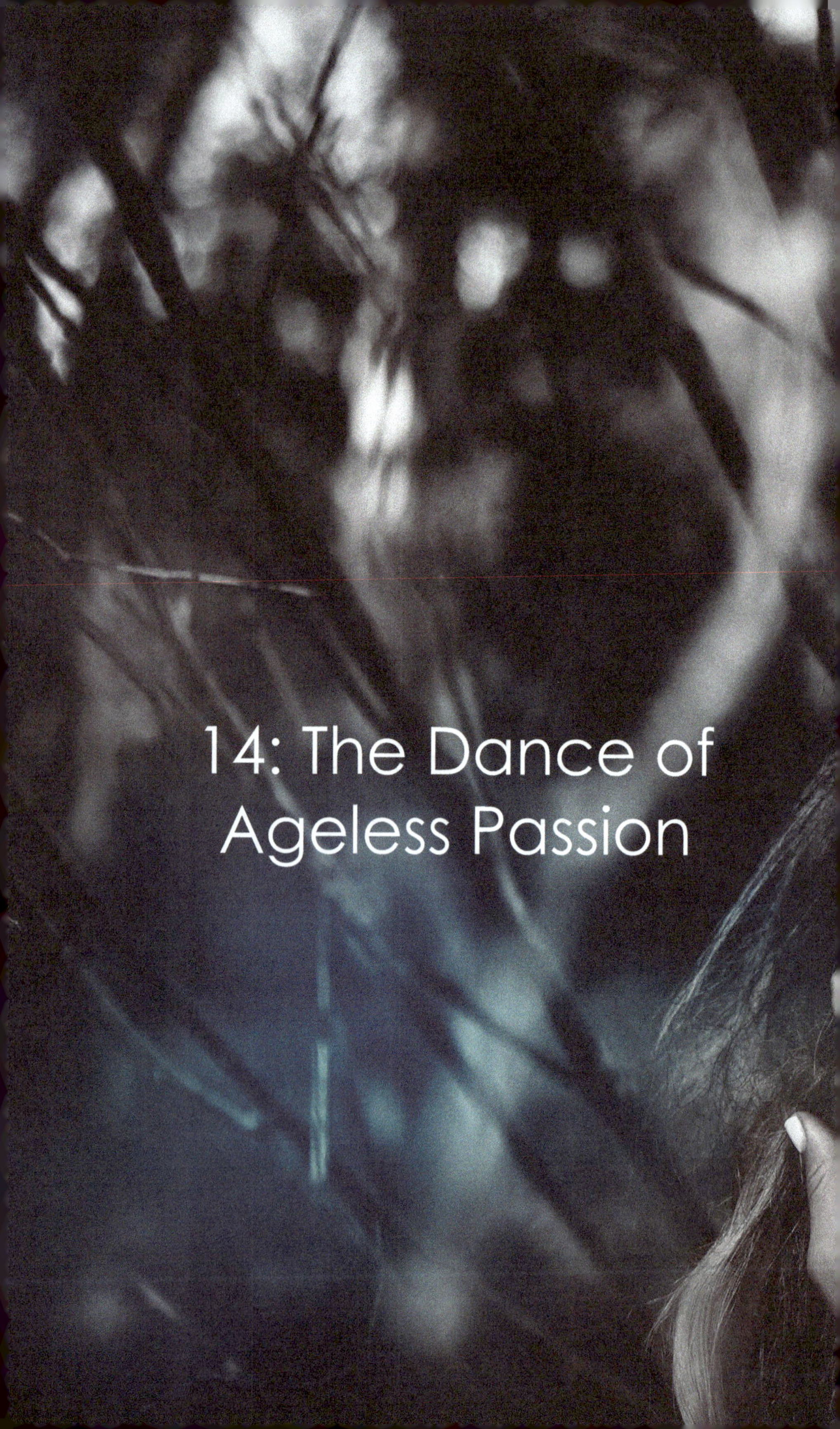

14: The Dance of Ageless Passion

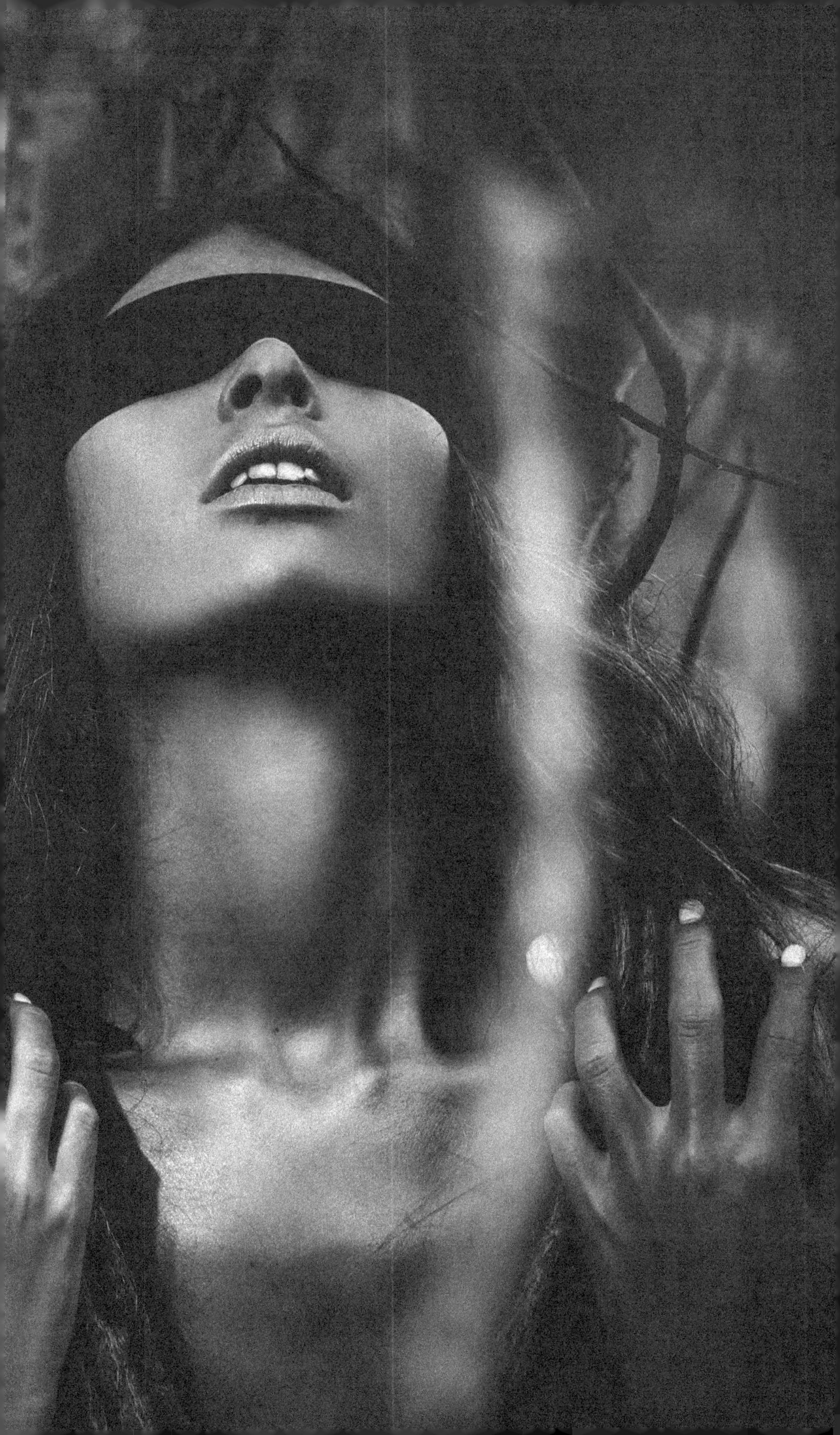

Chapter 14: The Dance of Ageless Passion

As Mia and Ethan journeyed into their early fifties, they entered a new season of their lives together. With each passing year, their bond had grown deeper, enriched by a tapestry of shared experiences. Yet, they also noticed the inevitable changes in their bodies, a natural progression that invited both adaptation and a renewed understanding.

Embracing these changes, they turned to the ancient wisdom of tantra, seeking to continue nurturing their intimate connection while honoring their evolving physical selves. It was in this spirit that they decided to explore a tantric ritual focused on enhancing orgasmic response, a practice adapted with reverence and curiosity to their changing bodies.

Transforming their bedroom into a sacred space, they dimmed the lights and lit fragrant incense, setting a serene and intimate atmosphere. Soft, ambient music played in the background, its melodies weaving through the room like a gentle caress.

Their ritual began with the creation of sacred space. Together, they set the intention for their practice, focusing on deepening intimacy and enhancing pleasure. This was not just a physical exploration, but a journey into the depths of their connection. Seated facing each other, they started with synchronized breathwork.
Inhaling and exhaling together, they found their energies aligning, their hearts syncing in a rhythm of shared life. Placing their hands over each other's hearts, they felt the steady beat beneath their palms, a testament to their enduring love and the life they had built together.

As they moved onto sensual touch and exploration, they lay down, taking turns to rediscover each other's bodies. Each touch was gentle and loving, an acknowledgment of how age had reshaped and redefined their physical forms. They communicated openly, guiding each other with kindness, exploring what felt good in this new phase of their lives.

The focus then shifted to the energy centers of their pleasure. Using a combination of light touches, breath, and visualization, they amplified sensations, creating a slow, deep arousal. This was different from the fiery passions of their youth but held a profound depth that resonated with their current selves.

Transitioning into more intimate touch, they maintained a mindful pace, deeply connected through gaze and breath. They explored each other, adapting to positions and movements that suited their bodies now, finding comfort and joy in this slower, more deliberate exploration of pleasure.

When they reached the culmination of their ritual, it was a powerful, resonant release. It was different from the intense peaks of their younger days, yet it held a deeper, more meaningful resonance. They experienced orgasm as a flowing wave of energy, a shared moment of joy and release.

Lying together in the afterglow, they shared their feelings and reflections, embracing the changes and discoveries made during their practice. They closed the ritual with gratitude for the journey they had shared and the new paths of pleasure and intimacy they were now exploring.

A Gentle Tantric Ritual

This practice is designed for intermediate - advanced tantric practitioners who wish to deepen their connection and explore higher levels of consciousness and intimacy. The focus is on subtlety, energy flow, and heightened awareness.

Total Duration: 45-60 minutes

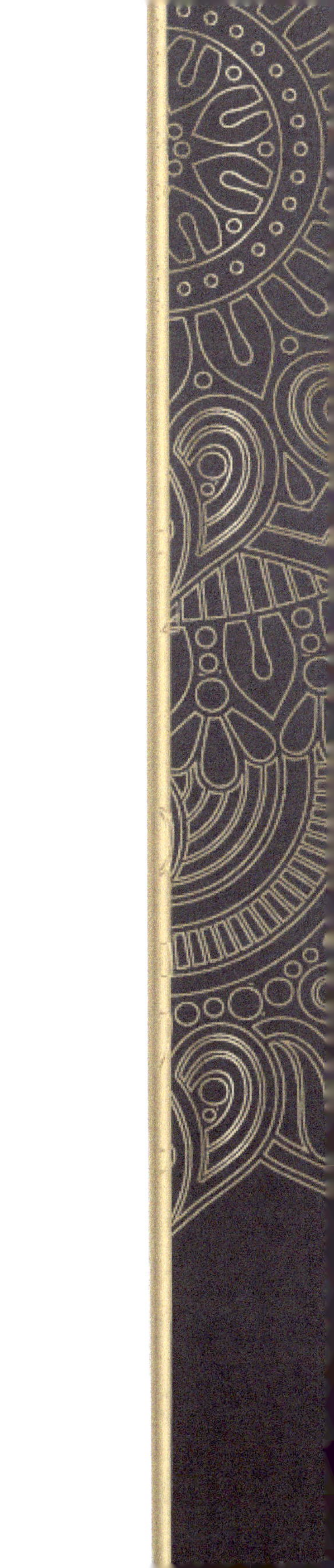

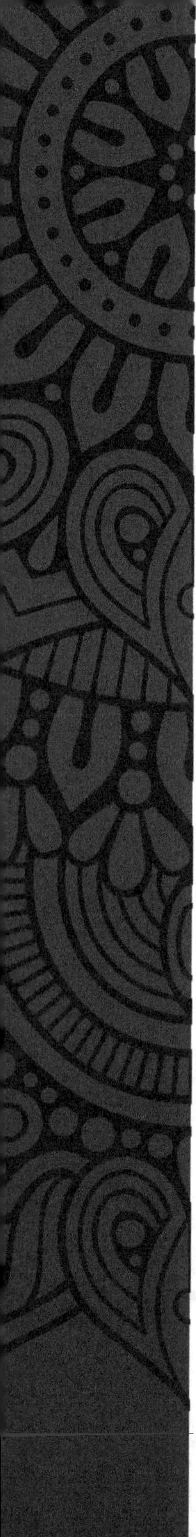

Preparation:
Create a Sacred and Intimate Space: Choose a quiet, comfortable area where you won't be disturbed. Decorate the space with elements that evoke tranquility and sacredness, like candles, flowers, or sacred objects.

Set the Ambiance: Play soft, ambient music or nature sounds to enhance the atmosphere. Ensure the room temperature is comfortable for both partners.

Grounding and Centering (5 minutes):
Joint Breathing: Sit facing each other, with your eyes closed, and begin by synchronizing your breathing. Inhale and exhale deeply together, establishing a shared rhythm and presence.

Energy Awakening (10 minutes):
Chakra Connection: With eyes still closed, visualize your chakras (energy centers) aligning with your partner's. Start from the root chakra, moving upward to the crown chakra. Imagine a stream of energy flowing between each of your chakras, connecting and balancing them.

Mantra Chanting: Silently chant a shared mantra (such as "Om" or a personal mantra) to harmonize your vibrations.

Subtle Touch Exploration (15 minutes):
Energy Sensing: Begin to explore each other's body with extremely light and gentle touches, almost hovering over the skin. Feel the energy radiating from each other's body without direct contact.

Synchronized Movement: Gradually introduce synchronized movements, like gentle swaying or rocking, to deepen the sense of connection and flow.

Intimate Gazing (10 minutes):
Eye Contact: Open your eyes and engage in soft, intimate eye gazing. Maintain a gentle, loving gaze, communicating

non-verbally and connecting deeply.

Silent Affirmation: Silently communicate love and appreciation through your eyes, deepening the emotional and spiritual bond.

Meditative Union (10 minutes):

Yab-Yum Position: If comfortable, assume the Yab-Yum position (one partner sitting on the other's lap) or a similar intimate position that allows close physical contact.

Breath and Energy Synchronisation: Continue to breathe in sync, visualising the energy circulating through and around both bodies, creating an aura of shared energy.

Closing the Practice (5 minutes):

Sharing Gratitude: Conclude the practice by expressing gratitude for each other and the shared experience.

Reflection: Sit in silence for a few moments, reflecting on the experience and the feelings of connectedness.

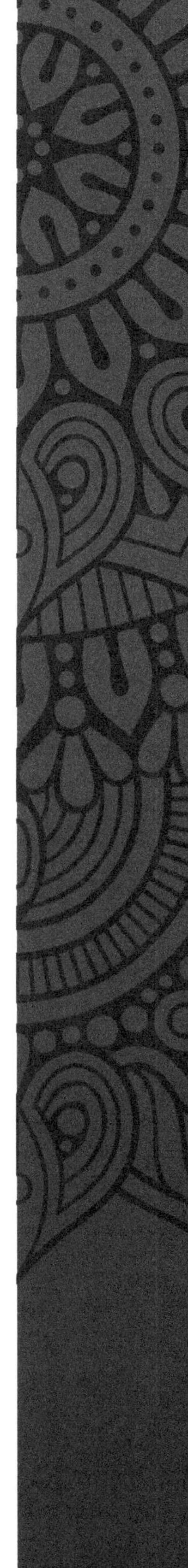

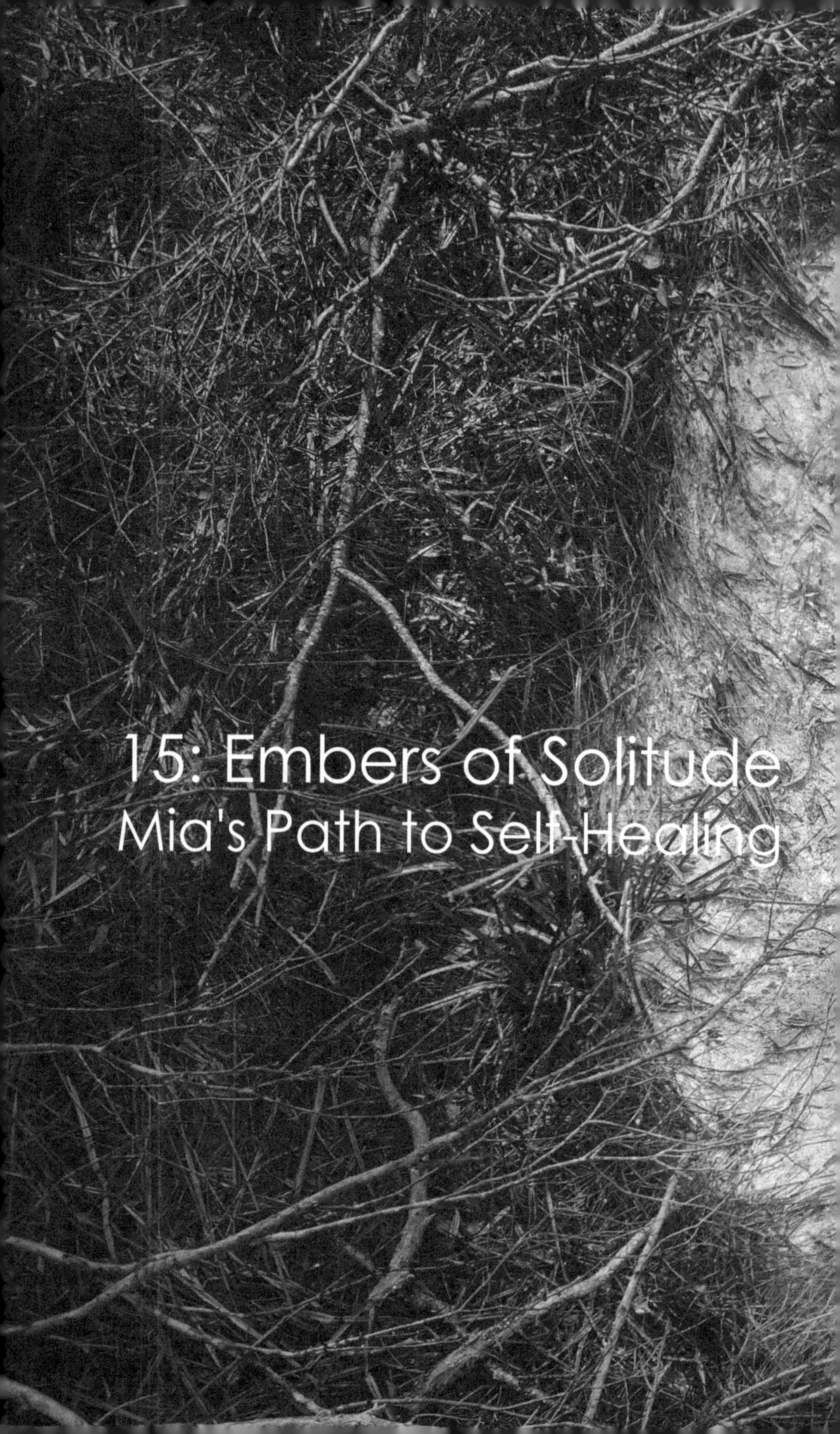
15: Embers of Solitude
Mia's Path to Self-Healing

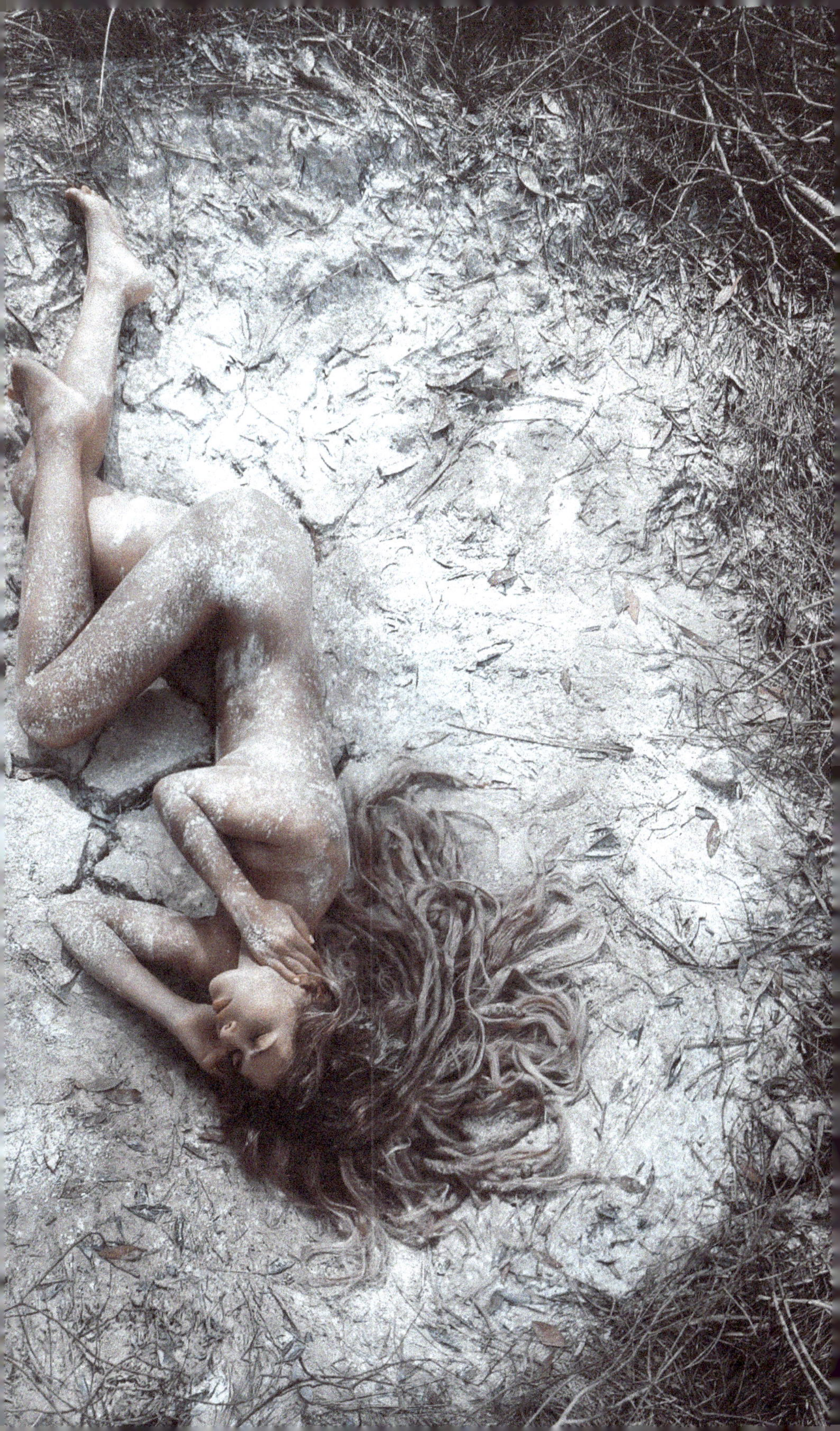

Chapter 15: Embers of Solitude: Mia's Path to Self-Healing

A little over a year had passed since Ethan left the earthly realm, leaving Mia in a world that felt quieter, emptier. Their cottage, once resonant with shared dreams and laughter, now echoed with the poignant memories of their deep, soulful connection.

Wrestling with her grief and the vast emptiness left behind, Mia found solace in the sacred practices of tantra, embracing them not only as a means of self-care but also as a way to keep the vibrant flame of passion and life burning within her, honoring the love and the profound lessons Ethan had imparted.

On a cool autumn evening, as the wind whispered secrets through the vineyards, Mia prepared for a personal tantric ritual. This ritual, a creation of her own design, was a blend of meditation, movement, and affirmation, intended to help her reconnect with her inner strength and vitality.
In her bedroom, now transformed into a sacred space with the gentle flicker of candles and the soothing scent of incense, Mia set her intention for the practice: to find healing, honor the enduring love within her heart, and reconnect with the essence of her being.

She began with deep, measured breaths, each inhale drawing in healing and strength, and each exhale releasing the tendrils of sorrow and loneliness. As she breathed, Mia visualized herself enfolded in a warm, golden light, a protective aura that nurtured her spirit.

Moving into a chakra meditation, Mia focused on each energy center, starting from the root and ascending upwards. She envisioned a vibrant energy coursing through her body, rejuvenating and balancing her physically and emotionally. This meditative journey through her chakras was a reminder of her own resilience and the continuous flow of life within her.

Rising to her feet, Mia allowed her body to sway and move freely to the rhythm of the soft, ambient music that filled the room. This dance was not one of structure or form but an expression of her innermost feelings – a dance of grief, love, longing, and the celebration of life. With each movement, she felt a reawakening, an affirmation of her enduring spirit.

Mia then settled back down for a session of self-massage, starting from her feet and working upwards. Each touch was a message of self-love and acceptance, acknowledging the journey her body had been through and its enduring strength. She paid attention to the areas that needed healing, each stroke a testament to her body's resilience.

As the ritual neared its end, Mia lay down and repeated affirmations of self-love and gratitude. She reflected on her journey with Ethan, smiling through the memories, allowing herself to feel the love that still permeated her being, and embracing her solitude as a space for growth and self-discovery.

Concluding the ritual, Mia felt a profound sense of peace and connection – to herself, to the essence of Ethan's spirit, and to the greater universe. As she extinguished the candles, she carried with her the warmth and energy from her practice.

Lying in bed in the stillness of the night, Mia felt a renewed sense of purpose and strength. The ritual had rekindled the eternal flame within her – a flame of passion, love, and life that Ethan had helped ignite and that she would continue to nurture. This path of self-care and self-love was not only a tribute to their shared life but also a testament to her own capacity for resilience and growth.

In her heart, she knew that this journey of self-healing was just beginning, a new chapter in her story of love and transformation.

Mia's Practice
for Self-Healing

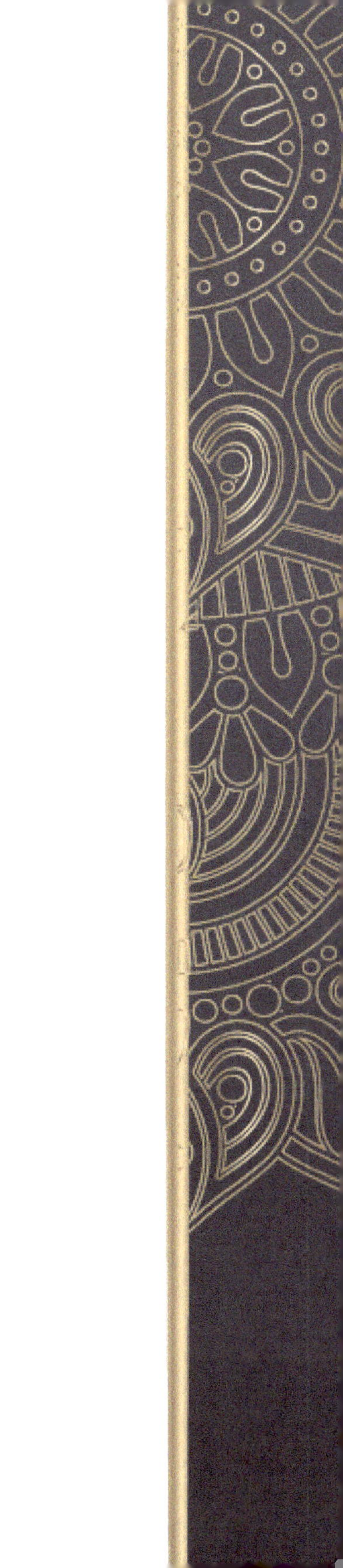

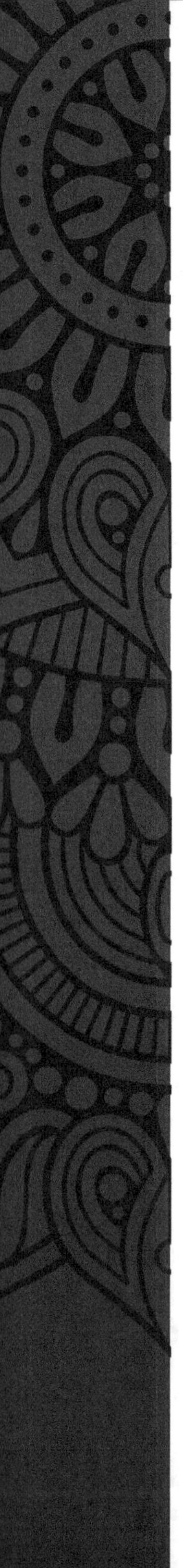

Preparation:
Create a Sacred Space: Mia transforms a quiet corner of her cottage into a sacred space.
She lays out a comfortable mat, lights candles for warmth and illumination and plays soft, soothing music to create a serene atmosphere.

Grounding and Centering (5 minutes):
Deep Breathing: Mia begins with deep, rhythmic breathing to center herself. She focuses on each inhale and exhale, allowing her breath to anchor her in the present moment.

Body Awareness: She gently shifts her focus through her body, acknowledging any sensations or emotions, and breathing into them with acceptance.

Heart Chakra Meditation (10 minutes):
Focus on the Heart: Mia places her hands over her heart, feeling its rhythm. She visualizes a green light at her heart center, symbolizing love, healing, and renewal.

Chanting: She softly chants the mantra "YAM," the sound vibration associated with the heart chakra, to open and balance this energy center.

Self-Compassion Exercise (5 minutes):
Affirmations: Mia speaks affirmations of self-love and acceptance, such as "I am whole," "I honor my journey," and "I embrace my strength and vulnerability."

Energy Flow Visualisation (10 minutes):
Visualize Healing Energy: Mia imagines a healing energy in the form of a warm, nurturing light that flows through her body. Starting from her crown and moving down to her toes, she visualises this light soothing and healing her body and spirit.

Connection with Nature: She visualises her energy connecting with the earth, feeling grounded and supported by nature's resilience and vitality.

Closing the Practice:
Gratitude and Reflection: Mia concludes the practice with
a moment of gratitude for her own strength, the memories
shared with Ethan, and the journey ahead.

Journaling: After the practice, she spends a few minutes
journaling her thoughts and reflections, allowing her to
process and integrate her experience.

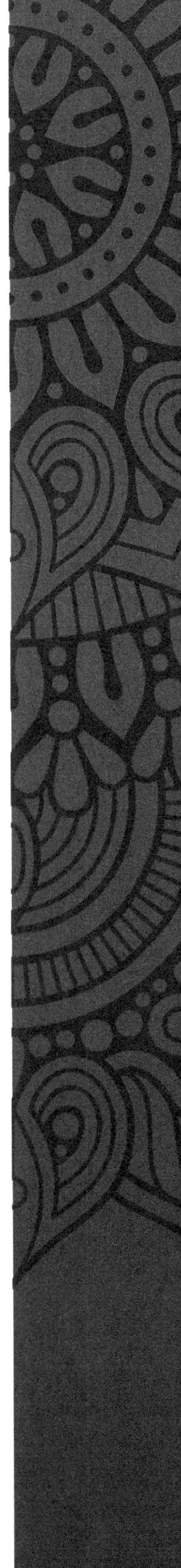

Eternal Flames

About the Author

COACH | SPEAKER | AUTHOR

Linda Ferrari is a mum, partner, sister, friend, feline fancier and garden dreamer.

Her mission, through the coaching practice, is to help people unlock their freedom and create a future they want, to act as a guide to reclaiming their lives, to thriving without compromising the important things.

www.lindaferrari.com.au